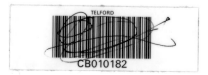

Dizziness, Hearing Loss, and Tinnitus

Dizziness, Hearing Loss, and Tinnitus

Robert W. Baloh, M.D.
Professor of Neurology and Surgery (Head and Neck)
Reed Neurological Research Center
University of California—Los Angeles
School of Medicine
Los Angeles, California

 F. A. DAVIS COMPANY • Philadelphia

F. A. Davis Company
1915 Arch Street
Philadelphia, PA 19103

Printed in the United States of America

Last digit indicates print number: 10 9 8 7 6 5 4 3 2 1

Acquisitions Editor: Robert W. Reinhardt
Developmental Editor: Bernice M. Wissler
Cover Designer: Louis J. Forgione

As new scientific information becomes available through basic and clinical research, recommended treatments and drug therapies undergo changes. The author(s) and publisher have done everything possible to make this book accurate, up to date, and in accord with accepted standards at the time of publication. The authors, editors, and publisher are not responsible for errors or omissions or for consequences from application of the book, and make no warranty, expressed or implied, in regard to the contents of the book. Any practice described in this book should be applied by the reader in accordance with professional standards of care used in regard to the unique circumstances that may apply in each situation. The reader is advised always to check product information (package inserts) for changes and new information regarding dose and contraindications before administering any drug. Caution is especially urged when using new or infrequently ordered drugs.

Library of Congress Cataloging in Publication Data

Baloh, Robert W. (Robert William), 1942–
   Dizziness, hearing loss, and tinnitus / Robert W. Baloh.
     p.   cm.
   Includes bibliographical references and index.
   ISBN 0-8036-0330-4 (hc : alk. paper)
   1. Deafness. 2. Dizziness. 3. Tinnitus. I. Title.
   [DNLM: 1. Vestibular Diseases. 2. Dizziness. 3. Hearing
Disorders. 4. Hearing Tests. 5. Vestibular Function Tests. WV
255 B195d 1998]
   RF290.B198 1998
   617.8′82—dc21
   DNLM/DLC
   for Library of Congress   97-42657
                                  CIP

This book is dedicated to Dr. Harold F. Schuknecht for his remarkable contributions to the field of neurotology.

Foreword

Dizziness, imbalance, tinnitus, and changes in hearing are common clinical complaints and, like all symptoms, demand a logical and thoughtful approach for successful diagnosis and management. Because these symptoms are frequently unaccompanied by obvious neurologic signs and are not perceived to be life-threatening, physicians often do not give them the attention they deserve. But these symptoms, even if not always disabling, are usually distracting and discomforting, and interfere with the quality of life. Accordingly, they do deserve attention and they need to be diagnosed properly and promptly, because they often can be successfully treated.

This book provides the needed information so that many types of physicians who see such patients—from family practitioners, emergency room physicians, and internists, to specialists in neurology, neurosurgery, and otolaryngology—will have a logical approach in mind for both the clinical history and physical examination and the subsequent laboratory evaluation. Particularly useful are the decision-making trees, used so frequently by Dr. Baloh, that guide the physician as to what tests to order and how far to go in the diagnostic workup of neurotologic symptoms. The book also provides practical information on treatment and presents the latest concepts on the more common conditions causing vertigo, including BPPV (benign paroxysmal positional vertigo), migraine, and transient ischemic attacks. Information on antibiotic ototoxicity and the genetic causes of dizziness is also presented.

But the Baloh approach is much more than a collection of recipes (albeit good ones) on how to do it. The book also provides the essential knowledge base of vestibular and auditory physiology and anatomy that allows one to diagnose the difficult cases and to detect and interpret the subtleties of the neurotologic history and examination. So this is an eminently practical guide, but one couched in scientific principles, allowing physicians to deal effectively with either the simple and straightforward or the rare and complex neurotologic case. Pervasive throughout this book is both the clinical experience and the basic fund of knowledge of the pre-eminent medical neurotologist in our country. Anyone who wants to get a handle on dizziness and hearing difficulties will benefit from reading this book.

David S. Zee, MD
Baltimore, Maryland

Preface

The purpose of this book is to present a concise, organized approach to evaluating patients who present with dizziness, hearing loss, and tinnitus. The book is divided into three parts: anatomy and physiology, history and examination, and diagnosis and treatment. In the first section, I briefly review clinically relevant anatomy and physiology to provide a framework for understanding the pathophysiology of vestibular and auditory symptoms. The second section outlines the important features in the patient's history and examination that determine the probable site of a lesion. Separate chapters provide a systematic approach to evaluating patients with different types of dizziness and different types of tinnitus. Numerous tables and flowcharts guide the reader through the diagnostic workup. Finally, the section on diagnosis and treatment covers the key differential diagnosis points that help the clinician decide on the cause of the patient's problem and how to treat it. The description of each disorder begins with an outline of symptoms, signs, laboratory findings, and treatment options. I included separate chapters on the symptomatic treatment of dizziness and tinnitus because one is often faced with treating these symptoms on an empirical basis.

I believe that this book will be useful to all physicians who deal with patients complaining of dizziness, hearing loss, and tinnitus. It can serve as an introduction to neurotology for students and resident physicians and as a practical reference source for practicing clinicians. It should be most helpful for those in the fields of family practice, internal medicine, neurology, audiology, otolaryngology, and neurosurgery. I have attempted to maintain a balanced presentation of otologic and neurologic disorders because I strongly believe that one cannot effectively evaluate neurotologic problems without understanding both the peripheral and central aspects of these disorders.

I want to acknowledge Bernice Wissler at F. A. Davis and Kate Jacobson at UCLA for their invaluable help in preparing this book. I also want to acknowledge the long-standing support of my work by the National Institutes of Health.

Robert W. Baloh

Contents

Part II
History and Examination

8. Approach to the Patient with Dizziness

9. Approach to the Patient with Tinnitus

Part III
Diagnosis and Treatment

Part I

Anatomy and Physiology

1

The Middle Ear

Chapter Outline

COMPONENTS

The middle ear consists of a series of irregular, pneumatic chambers within the temporal bone.[1] Three main chambers are routinely identified: the tympanic cavity, the mastoid antrum, and the eustachian tube (Fig. 1). The centrally located tympanic cavity, situated between the external and the internal ear, is traversed by a chain of small bones that transmit vibrations from the tympanic membrane to the labyrinth (Fig. 2). The **tympanic cavity** can be subdivided into a lower part corresponding in vertical extent to the tympanic membrane and an upper region extending above the upper border of the tympanic membrane, known as the epitympanic recess. The **mastoid antrum,** an irregular, bean-shaped cavity, communicates with the posterior epitympanic recess by an aperture, the aditus ad antrum. Many of the pneumatized spaces of the mastoid open directly into the antrum. Finally, the tympanic cavity communicates directly with the pharynx via the elongated **eustachian tube**.

DEVELOPMENT

In the embryo the middle ear develops from a pouch of the primitive gut, the first pharyngeal pouch.[2] As this pouch of entodermal origin moves toward the developing temporal bone, the mesenchymal tissue that fills the middle ear of the fetus recedes. Ciliated epithelium from the primitive gut covers the eustachian tube, tympanic cavity, and mastoid, forming an

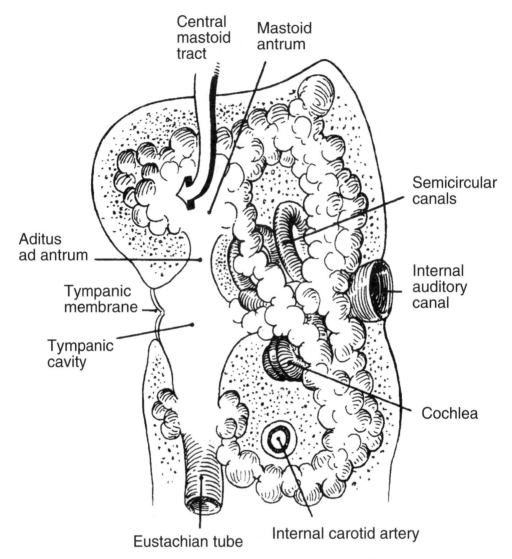

Central mastoid tract

Mastoid antrum

Semicircular canals

Aditus ad antrum

Internal auditory canal

Tympanic membrane

Tympanic cavity

Cochlea

Eustachian tube

Internal carotid artery

FIGURE 1   Schematic drawing of intercommunicating air cell system within the temporal bone. (Adapted from Schuknecht, HF: *Pathology of the Ear.* Harvard University Press, Cambridge, MA, 1974.)

The degree of pneumatization of the human temporal bone varies greatly. Passageways connecting the pneumatized spaces serve as routes for infection to spread through the bone from the middle ear.

endless variety of small cavities in a process known as **pneumatization** (see Fig. 1). The degree of pneumatization of the human temporal bone varies greatly, depending on hereditary factors, nutrition, and the adequacy of ventilation via the eustachian tube.[3] Each pneumatized space is usually in free communication with all other pneumatized spaces. Passageways that interconnect these air cells (e.g., the central mastoid tract indicated by the arrow in Fig. 1) serve as routes for infection to follow as it spreads from the middle ear through the temporal bone.

BOUNDARIES OF THE TYMPANIC CAVITY

The **lateral wall** of the tympanic cavity consists mainly of the tympanic membrane, together with the small rim of temporal bone to which it is attached. Superiorly, the lateral wall of the epitympanic recess is formed by the scutum, a plate of bone belonging to the squamous part of the temporal bone. The **medial wall** of the tympanic cavity is irregular, owing to several structures bulging from the inner ear: the promontory of the basal turn of the cochlea and the prominences of the facial canal and horizontal semicircular canal (see Fig. 2). The round window is located inferior and posterior to the promontory of the cochlea. This membrane seals the fluid in the scala tympani of the cochlea from the tympanic cavity. Posterior to the promontory is a smooth projection, the support of the promontory or the subiculum, that forms the inferior border of a deep depression known as the tympanic sinus. The oval window is located just above the promontory. It is closed by the stapes and the annular ligament.

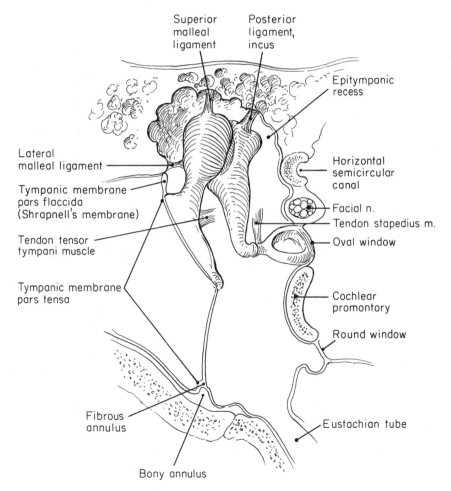

■ FIGURE 2   Cross section of the tympanic membrane and tympanic cavity.

The **anterior** or **carotid wall** of the tympanic cavity contains, from above to below, the insertion of the tensor tympani muscle, the orifice of the eustachian tube, and a thin, bony wall covered with air cells separating the tympanic cavity from the carotid canal. The **posterior** or **mastoid wall** contains the aditus ad antrum, an aperture transmitting the tendon of the stapedius muscle, a foramen by which the chorda tympani nerve enters the middle ear, and a fossa where the posterior ligament of the incus is attached.

The **roof** of the tympanic cavity is formed by the tegmen tympani, a thin plate of bone separating the epitympanic recess of the middle ear from the middle cranial fossa. The **floor** is very narrow transversely, being closely related to the fossa of the internal jugular vein. It is irregular, owing to the large number of air cells, and near the back there is a stylomastoid prominence corresponding to the root of the styloid process.

EUSTACHIAN TUBE

The eustachian tube connects the tympanic cavity with the nasopharynx, providing ventilation of the tympanic cavity and the adjacent pneumatized cavities of the temporal bone (see Figs. 1 and 2).[4] The tubal orifice at the nasopharynx is normally closed, but during deglutition it opens, owing to contraction of palate muscles that attach to the cartilage and elastic ligaments around the opening. The tensor veli palatini, the levator veli palatini, and the salpingopharyngeus muscles simultaneously contract during the act of swallowing or yawning, causing rotation and forceful pulling apart of the lateral and medial laminae of the eustachian tube cartilage. The tensor veli palatini, the most important of these muscles, is innervated by the mandibular division of the trigeminal nerve.

Failure of the eustachian tube to open during deglutition results in negative pressure in the pneumatized spaces of the temporal bone as a consequence of gases being absorbed into the blood stream. Improper opening of the eustachian tube may be due to an inflammatory reaction of the lining membrane such as occurs with infection or allergies of the upper respiratory tract. Other factors producing narrowing of the lumen include hyperplasia of lymphoid tissue, muscle weakness, neoplasia, and developmental anomalies such as those associated with cleft palate. Inadequate ventilative function of the eustachian tube in early life may inhibit pneumatization of the temporal bone and lead to chronic middle ear infections. Eustachian tube dysfunction is a major factor in the etiology of seromucinous otitis media.[4]

Eustachian tube dysfunction is a major factor in the etiology of seromucinous otitis media.

TYMPANIC MEMBRANE

The tympanic membrane consists of three layers: an inner mucosal layer, a middle fibrous layer, and an external epidermal layer.[5] It is conical in shape, with a diameter ranging from 8.5 to

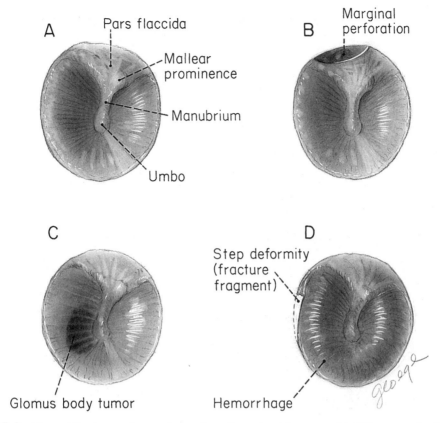

A   Pars flaccida

Mallear
prominence

Manubrium

Umbo

B   Marginal
perforation

C   Glomus body tumor

D   Step deformity
(fracture
fragment)

Hemorrhage

FIGURE 3   View of the tympanic membrane from the external ear canal in *(A)* a normal subject, and in patients with *(B)* a superior marginal perforation and cholesteatoma, *(C)* a tympanic glomus body tumor, and *(D)* a step deformity caused by a longitudinal temporal bone fracture. (From Baloh, RW and Honrubia, V: *Clinical Neurophysiology of the Vestibular System, ed. 2.* F.A. Davis, Philadelphia, 1990, p. 113, with permission.)

10 mm. From the external canal the tympanic membrane appears as a thin, semitransparent disc that normally has a glistening pearl-gray color (Fig. 3A). It is concave on its external surface, as if under traction from the manubrium of the malleus. The mallear stria (the manubrium shining through the tympanic membrane) passes from slightly inferior and posterior of the center (umbo) toward the superior margin of the tympanic membrane. Near the superior margin, the mallear prominence is formed by the lateral process of the malleus. From the mallear prominence, two folds stretch to the tympanic sulcus of the temporal bone, enclosing the triangular area of the pars flaccida, or Shrapnell's membrane. Rupture of the membrane at this site is commonly associated with invasion of the middle ear by keratinizing squamous epithelium from the external ear canal (Fig. 3B). This keratoma, or cholesteatoma, usually develops in the epitympanic space, from which it may extend posteriorly into the antrum and the central mastoid tract; inferiorly into the middle ear, where it may erode the ossicles and bony labyrinth; and superiorly into the intracranial cavity, producing central nervous system symptoms and

Rupture in the pars flaccida region of the tympanic membrane is commonly associated with invasion of the middle ear by keratinizing squamous epithelium (cholesteatoma) from the external ear canal.

Extension of cholesteatomas may erode the middle ear and produce central nervous system symptoms and signs.

signs. Lesions within the tympanic cavity often can be seen through the tympanic membrane because of its semitransparency (Figs. 3C and 3D).

THE OSSICULAR CHAIN

The ossicles provide an interface for transmitting to the inner ear changes in atmospheric pressure produced by sound waves. The long process of the **malleus**, the manubrium, is attached like the radius of a circle to the inner side of the tympanic membrane in a superoanterior direction (see Fig. 2). Superiorly, the head of the malleus is bound to the **incus**, forming the incudomalleal articulation, a type of diarthric joint. The long process of the incus directed downward and anteriorly is connected to the stapes, the smallest of the three middle ear ossicles. The footplate of the **stapes** articulates with the walls of the vestibule at the oval window, to which it is attached by a ring of ligaments. The dimensions of the window are 1.2×3 mm, with a total area that is one seventeenth that of the tympanic membrane. Sound-induced displacements of the tympanic membrane and its attached manubrium are transmitted through the medial arm of the assembly of middle ear bones acting as a lever to the inner ear; in this fashion the middle ear functions as a mechanical transformer. Additional amplification is produced as the force applied over the surface of the tympanic membrane is funneled into the smaller area of the oval window. The middle ear compensates for the loss of energy that would occur if sound were directly transmitted from air to the fluids of the inner ear. Without the middle ear structures, approximately 99.9% of the sound energy would be lost during this transmission.[6]

The ossicles are suspended by several ligaments and are dynamically controlled by the action of two muscles (see Fig. 2). The **tensor tympani,** innervated by a branch of the trigeminal nerve, is connected by a tendon into the upper part of the manubrium. Coursing in a lateral direction from the anterior part of the medial wall of the tympanic cavity, this muscle draws the manubrium medially, tensing the tympanic membrane. The **stapedius** muscle, innervated by the facial nerve, is attached to the posterior wall of the tympanic cavity and is directed anteriorly to anchor in the upper part of the stapes. Its contraction hinders the transmission of sound to the inner ear.

FACIAL NERVE

The facial nerve arises at the inferior border of the pons and proceeds to the internal auditory canal on the superior surface of the cochlear nerve. Within the temporal bone, four portions of the facial nerve can be classified (Fig. 4):

- The canal segment
- The labyrinthine segment
- The tympanic (horizontal) segment
- The mastoid (vertical) segment

The middle ear functions as a mechanical transformer, transmitting sound-induced displacements of the tympanic membrane to the inner ear.

Without the middle ear structures, about 99.9% of sound energy would be lost during transmission.

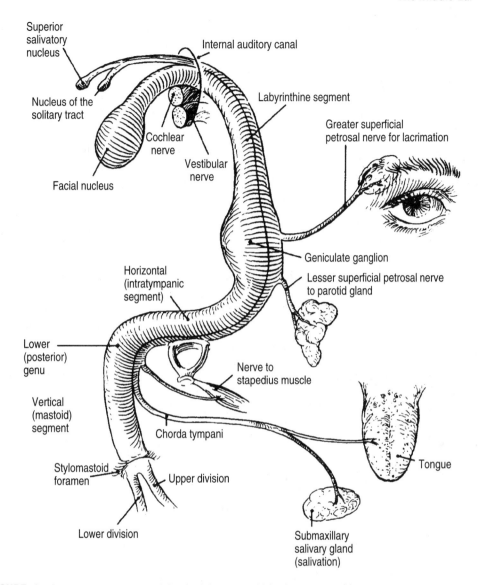

Superior
salivatory
nucleus

Internal auditory canal

Nucleus of the
solitary tract

Labyrinthine segment

Greater superficial
petrosal nerve for lacrimation

Cochlear
nerve

Vestibular
nerve

Facial nucleus

Geniculate ganglion

Horizontal
(intratympanic
segment)

Lesser superficial petrosal nerve
to parotid gland

Lower
(posterior)
genu

Nerve to
stapedius muscle

Vertical
(mastoid)
segment

Chorda tympani

Tongue

Stylomastoid
foramen

Upper division

Lower division

Submaxillary
salivary gland
(salivation)

■ **FIGURE 4**   Schematic diagram of the facial nerve within the temporal bone.

The **canal segment** runs in close company with the vestibular and cochlear divisions of the eighth nerve, while in its remaining segments the facial nerve lies separately within a bony canal—the facial, or fallopian, canal. The **labyrinthine segment** runs at nearly a right angle to the petrous pyramid, superior to the cochlea and vestibule, to reach the geniculate ganglion. At the geniculate ganglion the nerve takes a sharp turn posteriorly, marking the beginning of the tympanic segment. The **tympanic segment** passes along the medial wall of the tympanic cavity, superior to the oval window and inferior to the horizontal semicircular canal. At the sinus tympani the nerve bends inferiorly, marking the beginning of the **mastoid segment**. Four branches of the facial nerve lie within the temporal bone (see Fig. 4):

- The greater and the lesser superficial petrosal nerves, arising from the geniculate ganglion
- The nerve to the stapedius muscle, arising from the mastoid segment as it crosses the middle ear
- The chorda tympani, leaving the facial nerve approximately 5 mm above the stylomastoid foramen

The **greater superficial petrosal nerve** is composed of parasympathetic efferent fibers originating in the superior salivatory nucleus for innervation of the lacrimal glands and seromucous glands of the nasal cavity and of afferent cutaneous sensory fibers from parts of the external canal, tympanic membrane, and middle ear destined for the nucleus of the solitary tract. The **lesser superficial petrosal nerve** contains parasympathetic efferent fibers for the salivary glands. The **nerve to the stapedius muscle** and the main facial nerve trunk are motor nerves originating from the facial nucleus in the caudal pons. The **chorda tympani,** like the greater superficial petrosal, is a mixed nerve containing parasympathetic efferent fibers from the superior salivatory nucleus destined for the submaxillary glands and afferent taste fibers from the anterior two thirds of the tongue ending in the nucleus of the solitary tract.

Knowledge of the structure and function of each division of the facial nerve allows the clinician to localize lesions affecting the nerve within the temporal bone.

Knowledge of the structure and function of each division of the facial nerve allows the clinician to localize lesions affecting the nerve within the temporal bone.[7] Lesions in the internal auditory canal commonly involve both the seventh and the eighth cranial nerves. Lesions of the labyrinthine segment of the facial nerve above the geniculate ganglion impair ipsilateral

1. Lacrimation
2. Salivation
3. Stapedius reflex activity
4. Taste on the anterior two thirds of the tongue
5. Facial muscular strength

A lesion of the tympanic segment central to the nerve of the stapedius muscles affects only (3), (4), and (5) of the functions listed; and a lesion of the mastoid segment before the origin of the chorda tympani affects only (4) and (5); finally, a lesion at the stylomastoid foramen causes only ipsilateral facial muscle weakness or paralysis.

References

1. Anson BJ, and Donaldson AJ: Surgical Anatomy of the Temporal Bone, ed 3. W.B. Saunders, Philadelphia, 1981.
2. Anson BJ: Developmental anatomy of the ear. In Paparella MF, and Shumrick DA (eds): Otolaryngology, vol. 1. W.B. Saunders, Philadelphia, 1973.
3. Schuknecht HF: Pathology of the Ear. Lea & Febiger, Philadelphia, 1993.
4. Bluestone CD, Rood SR, and Swarts JD: Anatomy and physiology of the eustachian tube. In Cummings CW, et al (eds): Otolaryngology—Head and Neck Surgery, vol. 4. Mosby Year Book, St. Louis, 1993.

5. Duckert LG: Anatomy of the skull base, temporal bone, external ear, and middle ear. In Cummings CW, et al (eds): Otolaryngology — Head and Neck Surgery, vol. 4. Mosby Year Book, St. Louis, 1993.

6. Wever E, and Lawrence M: Physiological Acoustics. Princeton University Press, Princeton, 1954.

7. Dobie RA: Tests of facial nerve function. In Cummings CW, et al (eds): Otolaryngology — Head and Neck Surgery, vol. 4. Mosby Year Book, St. Louis, 1993.

2

The Inner Ear

Chapter Outline

PHYLOGENY OF THE LABYRINTH

The earliest gravity receptor organ, the statocyst, appeared more than 600 million years ago, in the late Precambrian era.[1] Beginning with primitive jellyfish, the statocyst allowed the animal to orient itself in relation to the horizon by sensing the direction of the gravitational force of the earth. The statocyst is a fluid-filled invagination, or sac, containing a calcinous particle, the statolith, or multiple particles, the statoconia, of density greater than the fluid. Attracted by gravity, the particles rest their weight differentially over special cells in the wall of the cyst. The direction of the force on the underlying sensory cells therefore depends on the position of the animal in space.

A continuous increment in anatomic complexity occurs in the evolution of the simple statocyst to the labyrinth of higher animals.[2] In primitive fish (cyclostomes), the statocyst cavity, previously open to the outside, is closed and filled by an endogenous secretion (endolymph). Two surviving cyclostomes, the hagfish and the lamprey, demonstrate an important step in the phylogenetic development of the vestibular labyrinth. In the hagfish, a simple circular tube is interrupted anteriorly and posteriorly by bulbous enlargements, the ampullae, each containing a primitive crista. Between the ampullae, in an intercommunicating channel, lies the macule communis, the forerunner of the utricular and saccular macules. The labyrinth of the lamprey is more complex, consisting of an anterior and a posterior canal communicating with a bilobulated sac containing separate utricular and saccular macules.

The predecessor of the cochlea appears after the development of a membranous labyrinth that is divided into two cavities.[3] In the inferior of the two cavities (the saccule), two new receptor areas develop, the lagenar macule and the basilar papilla. In amphibia, the basilar papilla is small compared with the lagena. In reptiles, a gradual enlargement of the basilar papilla occurs, so that in the crocodile the recess of the basilar papilla forms a long tube, the cochlear duct. The lagena in crocodiles and birds is displaced into a widened blind sac forming the end of the cochlear duct. The curvature of the cochlear duct is slight in birds but is much more pronounced in mammals, where a varying number of coils form a complete cochlea. The basilar membrane first appears in the reptilian stage of evolution. The sensory epithelium of the basilar membrane forms the basilar papilla in birds and the organ of Corti in mammals.

DEVELOPMENT OF THE LABYRINTH

In the embryo, the membranous labyrinth begins as ectodermal thickenings, the otic placodes, on each side of the rhombencephalon (Fig. 5).[4] The primitive otocyst forms by invagination of the otic placode, which becomes the inner layer of the membranous labyrinth. Three primary components develop through infolding of the walls of the otocyst:

- The endolymphatic duct and sac
- The utricle and semicircular canals
- The saccule and cochlear duct

The walls of the membranous labyrinth consist of an inner layer of ectodermal origin and an outer layer of mesodermal origin separated by a basement membrane. Regions of the inner layer subsequently develop into the specialized sensory organs.

It is helpful to know the interrelationships and timing of the development of the different inner ear structures, since congenital developmental defects can occur at each stage of development. The inner ear begins to develop approximately 3 weeks after conception with the appearance of the placodes. The placode rapidly forms the otocyst, and invagination within the vesicular wall divides it into vestibular and cochlear components (Fig. 5A–C). Concurrent with placode-otocyst development, the statoacousticofacial ganglion forms from the neural crest at the end of the third week. The otocyst develops into the vestibular duct, from which an anteroinferior cochlear diverticulum develops (Fig. 5D). By the end of the fourth week of development, the vestibular duct differentiates into the three semicircular canals as the cochlear duct begins to develop from its

The inner ear begins to develop approximately 3 weeks after conception.

By the end of the fourth week, the vestibular duct differentiates into three semicircular canals as the cochlear duct begins to develop.

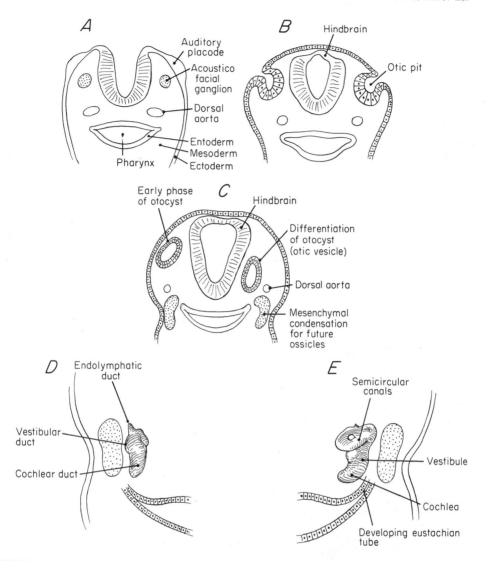

FIGURE 5 Embryologic development of the ear: (*A*) auditory placode stage, (*B*) otic pit stage, (*C*) otocyst-otic vesicle development, (*D*) and (*E*) labyrinthine development. (Adapted from Pearson, AA: *The Development of the Ear: A Manual.* American Academy of Ophthalmology and Otolaryngology, Rochester, MN, 1967.)

inferior, saccular portion (Fig. 5E). The cochlear turns begin to form by the sixth to seventh week, with completion of two and one-half turns by the eighth week. By the fifth month, the primitive organ of Corti has formed within the cochlear duct. The statoacousticofacial ganglion divides into a superior portion that sends fibers to the utricle and ampullae of the anterior and horizontal semicircular canals and into an inferior portion that sends fibers to the saccule and ampulla of the posterior semicircular canal. The remainder of the acoustic ganglion becomes the spiral ganglion of the cochlea.

By the fifth month, the primitive organ of Corti is formed within the cochlear duct.

FLUID DYNAMICS OF THE INNER EAR

The **bony labyrinth** is a series of hollow channels within the petrous portion of the temporal bone (Fig. 6). It consists of an anterior cochlear part, a posterior vestibular part, and a central chamber, the vestibule. Medial to the bony labyrinth is the **internal auditory canal**, a cul-de-sac housing cranial nerves VII and VIII and the internal auditory artery. The aperture on the cranial side is located at approximately the center of the posterior face of the pyramid of the temporal bone. Two other important orifices are in this vicinity. Halfway between the opening of the internal auditory canal and the sigmoid sinus, the slitlike aperture of the **vestibular aqueduct** contains the **endolymphatic sac**, a structure important in the exchange of endolymph. The second opening is that of the **cochlear aqueduct**, at the same level as the internal auditory canal but on the inferior side of the pyramid. The labyrinthine opening of this channel is located in the scala tympani, providing a connection between the subarachnoid and the

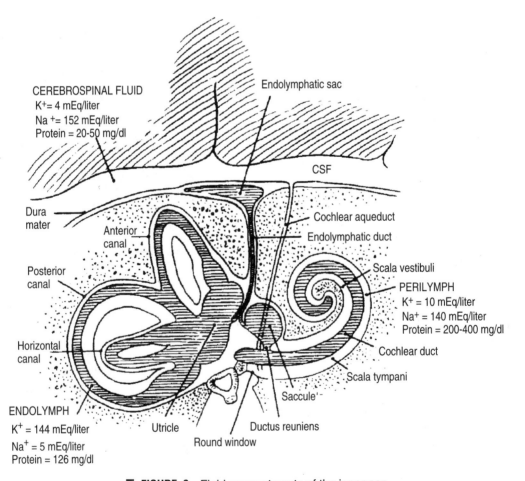

FIGURE 6   Fluid compartments of the inner ear.

perilymphatic spaces. The **membranous labyrinth** is enclosed within the channels of the bony labyrinth. A space containing perilymphatic fluid, a supportive network of connective tissue and blood vessels, lies between the periosteum of the bony labyrinth and the membranous labyrinth; the spaces within the membranous labyrinth contain endolymphatic fluid.

Perilymph is primarily formed by filtration from blood vessels in the inner ear.[5] As indicated previously, perilymph communicates with the cerebrospinal fluid (CSF) through the cochlear aqueduct, a narrow channel 3 to 4 mm long, with its inner ear opening at the base of the scala tympani (see Fig. 6). In most instances this channel is filled by a loose net of fibrous tissue continuous with the arachnoid. The size of the bony canal varies from individual to individual. Infection and blood within the CSF can make their way to the inner ear via the cochlear aqueduct.

The most likely site for production of endolymph is the secretory cells in the stria vascularis of the cochlea and the dark cells of the vestibular labyrinth.[5] It is generally agreed that resorption of endolymph takes place in the endolymphatic sac (see Fig. 6). Dye and pigment injected experimentally into the cochlea of animals accumulate in the endolymphatic sac; electron microscopic studies of the lining membrane of the sac reveal active pinocytotic activity.[6] Destruction of the epithelium lining the sac, or occlusion of the duct, results in an increase of endolymphatic volume in experimental animals.[7] The first change is an expansion of cochlear and saccular membranes that may completely fill the perilymphatic spaces. The anatomical changes resulting from this experiment are comparable to those found in the temporal bones of patients with Ménière's disease (either idiopathic or secondary to known inflammatory disease) (see Fig. 71).

The chemical composition of the fluids filling the inner ear is similar to that of the extracellular and intracellular fluids throughout the body.[5] The endolymphatic system contains intracellular-like fluids with a high potassium and a low sodium concentration, whereas the perilymphatic fluid resembles the extracellular fluids, having a low potassium and a high sodium concentration (see Fig. 6).[8] The endolymphatic sac has a much higher protein content than does the endolymphatic space, consistent with its role in the resorption of endolymph. The electrolyte composition of the endolymph and perilymph is critical for normal functioning of the sensory organs bathed in fluid. Ruptures of the membranous labyrinth in experimental animals cause destruction of the sensory and neural structures at the site of the endolymph-perilymph fistula.[9] Spontaneous ruptures of the membranous labyrinth may be the cause of episodic symptoms in patients with Ménière's disease. With the rupture, potassium leaks from the endolymph to the perilymph, inhibiting the bioelectric activity of the cochlear and vestibular hair cells. The potassium is then slowly cleared from the perilymph, and labyrinthine function returns to normal within 2 to 3 hours (a typical duration of an attack in Ménière's disease).

Infection and blood within the CSF can reach the inner ear via the cochlear aqueduct.

Destruction of the epithelial lining of the endolymphatic sac or occlusion of the endolymphatic duct results in an increase in endolymphatic volume and in endolymphatic hydrops in experimental animals.

Spontaneous ruptures of the membranous labyrinth may be the cause of episodic symptoms in patients with Ménière's disease.

BLOOD SUPPLY OF THE INNER EAR

The artery that supplies the membranous labyrinth and its neural structures is a branch of an intracranial vessel and does not communicate with arteries in the otic capsule and the middle ear.[6,10] This vessel, the **internal auditory** or **labyrinthine artery**, usually originates from the anterior inferior cerebellar artery, but exceptionally it arises directly from the basilar artery or some of its branches (Fig. 7; see also Figs. 62 and 64). As it enters the temporal bone, it forms branches that irrigate the ganglion cells, nerves, dura, and arachnoid membranes in the internal auditory canal. Shortly after entering the inner ear, the labyrinthine artery divides into two main branches, the **common cochlear artery** and the **anterior vestibular artery**. Because the arteries course independently, occlusion of one branch can result in selective damage to one part of the labyrinth. The common cochlear artery forms two branches, the posterior vestibular artery and the main cochlear artery. The latter enters the central canal of the cochlea, where it generates the radiating arterioles, forming a plexus within the cochlea irrigating the spiral ganglion, the structures in the basilar membrane, and the stria vascularis. The posterior vestibular artery, a branch from the common cochlear artery, is the source of blood supply to the inferior part of the saccule and the ampulla of the posterior semicircular canal. The other primary branch of the labyrinthine artery, the anterior vestibular artery, provides irrigation to the utricle and ampulla of the anterior and horizontal semicircular canals, as well as some blood to a small portion of the saccule.

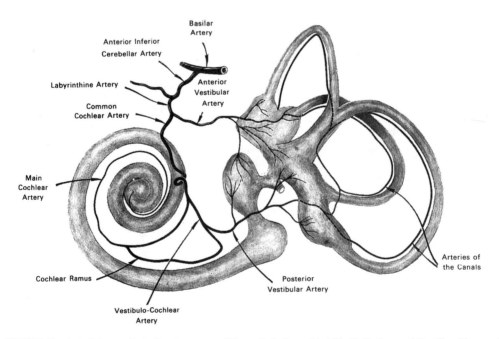

FIGURE 7   Arterial supply to the inner ear. (From Schuknecht, HF: *Pathology of the Ear.* Harvard University Press, Cambridge, MA, 1974, with permission.)

Interruption of the blood supply in the internal auditory artery or any of its branches seriously impairs the function of the inner ear, since the labyrinthine arteries do not anastomose with any other major arterial branch.[6,11] Within 15 seconds of blood flow interruption, the auditory nerve fibers become unexcitable, and the receptor and resting potentials in the ear abruptly diminish. If the interruption lasts for a prolonged period, the changes are irreversible; loss of function is followed by degenerative changes wherein ganglion cells and sensory cells undergo autolysis and new bone growth fills the ear cavity.

Interruption of the blood supply in the internal auditory artery or any of its branches seriously impairs the function of the inner ear, because the labyrinthine arteries do not anastomose with any other major arterial branch.

THE HAIR CELL

The basic element of the inner ear that transduces the mechanical forces associated with sound and head acceleration to nerve action potentials is the hair cell.[12] Two types of hair cells occur in birds and mammals (Fig. 8). Type II cells are cylindrical, with multiple nerve terminals at their base, whereas type I cells are globular or flask-shaped, with a single large, chalicelike nerve terminal surrounding the base. A bundle of nonmobile **stereocilia** protrudes from the cuticular plate on the apical end of each receptor cell. The height of the stereocilia increases stepwise from one side to the other, and next to the tallest stereocilia a thicker, longer hair, the **kinocilium**, protrudes from the cell's cytoplasm through a segment of cell membrane lacking the cuticular plate. Hair cells in the cochlea have only a rudimentary kinocilium.

The adequate stimulus for hair cell activation is a force acting parallel to the top of the cell, resulting in bending of the hairs (a shearing force).[13] A force applied perpendicular to the cell surface (a compressional force) is ineffective in stimulating the hair cell. The stimulus is maximal when the force is directed along an axis that bisects the bundle of stereocilia and goes through the kinocilium. Deflection of the hairs toward the kinocilium decreases the resting membrane potential of the sensory cells (depolarization). Bending in the opposite direction produces the reverse effect (hyperpolarization).

The adequate stimulus for hair cell activation is a force acting parallel to the top of the cell, bending the hairs (a shearing force).

Most of the basic information regarding the physiological properties of hair cells and their afferent nerves has been obtained through a study of hair cell systems in nonmammalian species.[14] Analysis of the lateral line organs of fish and amphibians has been particularly useful. These organs consist of groups of hair cells, the neuromasts, aligned in longitudinal rows on the side of the animal's body and head. A free-standing gelatinous cupula covering the hairs transmits the force associated with water displacement into hair cell deflection, which in turn results in a change in firing rate of the afferent nerve. The afferent nerves from lateral line organs generate continuous spontaneous activity. This observation has subsequently been confirmed in all other hair cell systems and represents a fundamental discovery in sensory physiology. Although the mechanism responsible for the spontaneous firing of action potentials in the afferent nerves has

The afferent nerves from the inner ear generate continuous spontaneous activity. Bending the hairs toward the kinocilium increases the spontaneous firing rate, and bending the hairs away from the kinocilium decreases it.

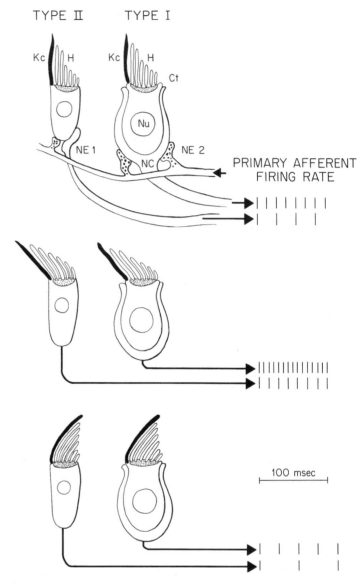

FIGURE 8 Hair cell modulation of spontaneous afferent nerve firing rate. Bending of the stereocilia toward the kinocilium depolarizes the hair cell and increases the firing rate, and bending away from the kinocilium hyperpolarizes the hair cell and decreases the firing rate. Kc = kinocilium, H = hairs, Ct = cuticular plate, Nu = nucleus, NC = nerve chalice, NE = nerve ending (1 = afferent, 2 = efferent).

not been identified, depolarization and hyperpolarization of the hair cells' membrane potential result in a modulation of this spontaneous activity (see Fig. 8). Bending of the hairs toward the kinocilium results in an increase of the spontaneous firing rate, and bending of the hairs away from the kinocilium results in a decrease. The spontaneous firing rate varies among different animal species and among different sensory receptors. It is thought to be greatest in the afferent neurons of the semicircular canals of mammals (up to 90 spikes per second) and lowest in some of the acoustic nerve fibers innervating mammalian cochlear hair cells (1 to 2 spikes per second).

Hair cells are not passive elements; they actively participate in the transduction process.[15] The stereocilia contain contractile proteins and can vary their length and stiffness under direct electrical stimulation. Thus the mechanical properties of hair cells can be influenced by the electrical currents of neighboring physiologically activated cells and by postsynaptic potentials from efferent neurons.[16]

THE INNER EAR RECEPTOR ORGANS

In the vestibular labyrinth the hair cells are mounted in the macules and the cristae, and in the cochlea, they are mounted in the organ of Corti. The hair cells function in the same way (as described previously) in each of these organs, yet the biological signals generated are quite different. This difference is due to the mechanical properties of the supporting structures.

The Macule

The membranous labyrinth forms two globular cavities within the vestibule, the **utricle** and the **saccule** (see Figs. 6 and 7). Each cavity contains a separate **macule**. In the saccule, the macule is located on the medial wall in the sagittal plane; in the utricle, the macule is primarily in the horizontal plane next to the opening of the horizontal semicircular canal (Fig. 9C). The surfaces of the utricular and saccular macules are covered by the **otolithic membrane**, a structure consisting of a mesh of fibers embedded in a gel with a superficial layer of calcium carbonate crystals, the **otoconia** (Fig. 9A). The stereocilia of the macular hair cells protrude into the otolithic membrane. The **striola**, a distinctive curved zone running through the center, divides each macule into two areas. The hair cells on each side of the striola are oriented so that their kinocilia are in opposite directions (as indicated by arrows in Fig. 9C). In the utricle, the kinocilia face the striola, and in the saccule, they face away from it. Because of this different orientation, displacement of the otolithic membrane has an opposite physiological influence on the set of hair cells on each side of the striola.

The density of the otolithic membrane overlying the hair cells of the macules is much greater than that of the surrounding endolymph, owing to the presence of the calcium carbonate crystals. The weight of this membrane produces a shearing force on the underlying hair cells that is proportional to the sine of the angle between the line of gravitational force and a line perpendicular to the plane of the macule (Fig. 9B). During

The density of the otolithic membrane overlying the hair cells of the macules is much greater than that of the surrounding endolymph, owing to the presence of calcium carbonate crystals.

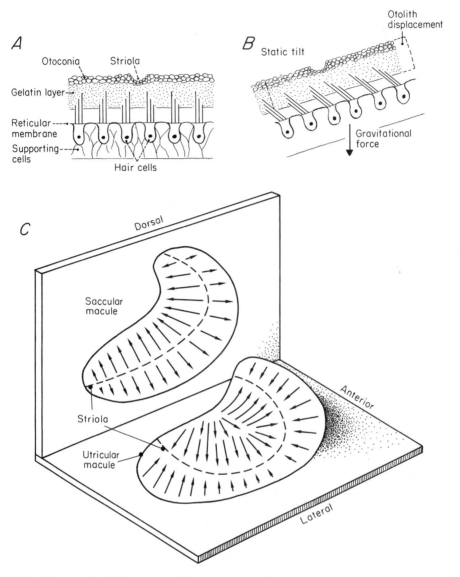

FIGURE 9 The macule: (*A*) anatomy, (*B*) mechanism of hair cell activation with static tilt, and (*C*) spatial orientation of saccular and utricular macules. Arrows indicate the direction that the kinocilia point toward. (Adapted from Barber, HO and Stockwell, CW: *Manual of Electronystagmography.* CV Mosby Co., St. Louis, 1976.)

linear head acceleration tangential to the surface of the receptor, the force acting on the hair cells is the result of two vector forces: one in the opposite direction of the head displacement and the other in the direction of gravitational pull. Recordings of afferent neuronal activity from the macules of primates confirm that the utricular and saccular macules are responsive to static tilt and dynamic linear acceleration forces.[17-20] The pattern of afferent nerve response is complex, however, with different neurons exhibiting different resting activity, frequency response, and adaptation properties.

The Crista

The **semicircular canals** are aligned to form a coordinate system. The horizontal canal makes a 30° angle with a horizontal plane, and the vertical canals make a 45° angle with a frontal plane (Fig. 10C).[21] At the anterior opening of the horizontal and anterior semicircular canals and the inferior opening of the posterior semicircular canal, each tube enlarges to form the **ampulla** (see Figs. 6 and 7). The crista, the sensory epithelium composed of hair cells and supporting cells, crosses each ampulla in a direction perpendicular to the longitudinal axis of the canal (Fig. 10A). Hair cells are located on the surface of the crista, with their cilia protruding into the **cupula**, a gelatinous mass of the same composition as the otolithic membrane. The cupula extends from the surface of the crista to the ceiling of the ampulla, forming what appears to be a watertight seal.

The hair cells within each crista are oriented with their kinocilia in the same direction.[22] In the horizontal canal, however, the kinocilia are directed toward the utricular side of the ampulla (as in Fig. 10A and B), whereas in the vertical canals the kinocilia are directed toward the canal side of the ampulla. This difference in morphological polarization explains the difference in directional sensitivity between the horizontal and the vertical canals. The afferent nerve fibers of the horizontal canals increase their baseline firing rate when endolymph moves toward the utricle or ampulla (ampullopetal flow), but the afferent nerve fibers of the vertical canals increase their baseline firing rate with endolymph flow away from the ampulla (ampullofugal flow).

Since the cupula has the same specific gravity as the surrounding fluids, it is not subject to displacement by changes in the line of gravitational force. The forces associated with angular head acceleration displace the cupula and bend the hair cells of the crista, however (Fig. 10B). The motion of the cupula can be likened to that of a pendulum in a viscous medium. Sudden displacement of the cupula by a step of angular head acceleration is followed by a gradual exponential return of the cupula to its baseline position. The rate of return is determined by the ratio of the viscous drag coefficient of the endolymph to the elasticity coefficient of the cupula according to the so-called torsion-pendulum model.[16]

Precise measurements of primary afferent nerve activity originating from the cristae of squirrel monkeys during physiological rotatory stimulation reveal that the change in frequency of action potentials is approximately proportional to the deviation of the cupula as predicted by the torsion-pendulum model.[23-25] For example, during sinusoidal head rotation in the plane of a semicircular canal, a sinusoidal change in firing frequency is superimposed on a rather high resting discharge (about 90 spikes per second) (Fig. 11). The peak firing rate occurs at the time of maximum cupular displacement, which occurs at the time of peak angular head velocity. With small-amplitude sinusoidal rotation, the modulation is almost symmetrical about the baseline firing rate. For larger stimulus amplitudes, the responses become increas-

The hair cells within each crista are oriented with their kinocilia in the same direction; in the horizontal canal the kinocilia are directed toward the utricular side of the ampulla, and in the vertical canals the kinocilia are directed toward the canal side of the ampulla.

The cupula moves like a pendulum in a viscous medium. Sudden displacement of the cupula by a step of angular head acceleration is followed by a gradual exponential return to its baseline position.

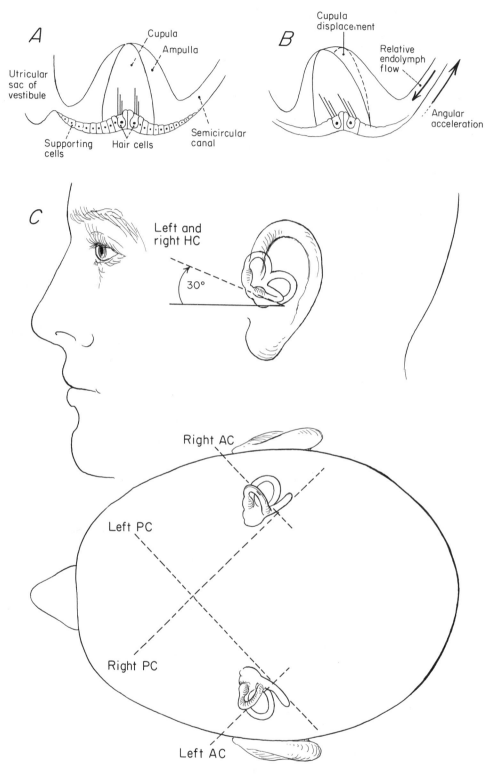

FIGURE 10   The crista: (*A*) anatomy, (*B*) mechanism of hair cell activation with angular acceleration, and (*C*) orientation of the semicircular canals within the head. HC = horizontal canal,
PC = posterior canal, AC = anterior canal.

Angular Head
Velocity

Cupular
Displacement

Afferent Nerve
Firing Rate

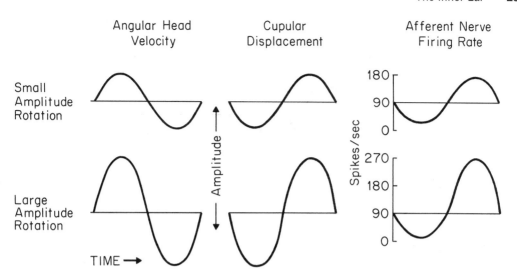

FIGURE 11   Relationship between angular head velocity, cupular displacement, and primary afferent nerve firing rate during sinusoidal angular rotation in the plane of the horizontal semicircular canal. During small-amplitude rotation the modulation of afferent nerve activity is approximately symmetrical about the baseline level (approximately 90 spikes per second), whereas with large-amplitude rotation the modulation is markedly asymmetric.

ingly asymmetrical. The excitatory responses can increase to as many as 350 to 400 spikes per second in proportion to stimulus magnitude, whereas the growth of inhibitory response is limited to the disappearance of spontaneous activity. This asymmetry in afferent nerve response partially explains why rotation-induced nystagmus is asymmetrical in patients with only one functioning labyrinth (see Rotational Testing in Chapter 6).

The Organ of Corti

The **cochlear duct** is a spiral membranous canal that subdivides the bony spiral canal of the cochlea into the scala vestibuli and scala tympani (Fig. 12C)[26]. The spiral ligament, located in a sulcus on the external wall of the bony cochlear duct, serves as the external attachment of the basilar membrane and Reissner's membrane. The scala media, between Reissner's membrane and the basilar membrane, contains endolymph; the scala vestibuli and scala tympani contain perilymph (see Fig. 6). The **organ of Corti** is mounted on the scala media side of the basement membrane.

Hair cells in the organ of Corti contain only stereocilia, being devoid of kinocilia. The stereocilia project into the **tectorial membrane**, a gelatinous structure overlying the organ of Corti. The ends of the cilia rest within pockets in the tectorial membrane. Upward displacement of the basilar membrane results in a shearing force between the organ of Corti and the tectorial membrane. The hair cells are displaced in relation to the relatively fixed tectorial membrane (acting as a hinge) (Fig. 12B).

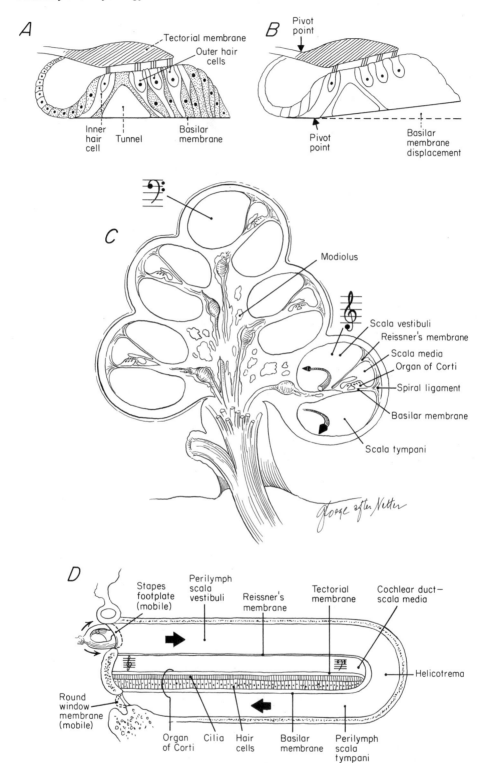

FIGURE 12 The organ of Corti: (*A*) anatomy, (*B*) mechanism of hair cell activation with sound-induced basilar membrane displacement, (*C*) and (*D*) direction of fluid displacement within the cochlea. In (*D*) the spiral cochlea has been schematically unwound. Arrows indicate direction of perilymph movement. The bass clef (top) and treble clef (middle) shown in *C* indicate where these sounds are located on the cochlea.

Inward movement of the stapes displaces the inner ear fluid toward the round window, resulting in outward movement of the round window membrane (Fig. 12D). This movement of fluid sets into motion a complicated wave form on the basilar membrane, exciting the hair cells of the organ of Corti as just described.[27,28] According to the traveling wave theory, maximum displacement of the basement membrane occurs at different distances from the stapes depending on the frequency of the sound. For low-frequency sounds maximum displacement occurs near the apex, but for high-frequency sounds maximum displacement is closer to the base. Measurements of action potentials from single acoustic nerve fibers reveal a frequency-dependent excitability that resembles the filter properties of the basilar membrane. Each fiber has a characteristic frequency at which it is most sensitive. The sensitivity decays very rapidly for frequencies on either side of this characteristic frequency.

Since frequency has a spatial distribution within the cochlea, lesions involving restricted areas of the cochlea are expressed functionally as threshold losses for different parts of the auditory spectrum. In animals, surgically induced lesions in the apical region cause hearing loss for low frequencies, whereas lesions of the basal end of the cochlea create severe high-frequency hearing losses.[29] Clinical-pathological studies in patients with hearing loss have documented a similar frequency-spatial distribution within the human cochlea (see Fig. 79).

Unifying Concept of Hair Cell Function

In all cases, the effective stimulus to the sensory cells in the labyrinth is the relative displacement of the cilia produced by application of mechanical force to the cilia's surroundings. Since the mechanical properties of the "supporting and coupling" structures are different, the frequency ranges at which the cilia can be moved by the applied force also are different. The otolithic membrane is maximally displaced during constant linear acceleration such as that associated with gravity, but its motion rapidly diminishes if the linear acceleration changes at a frequency greater than 0.5 Hz, owing to the characteristics of the restraining viscoelastic forces holding the otolith to the macule. The semicircular canals respond only to angular acceleration at frequencies below 5 Hz, owing to the inertial and viscous forces restraining the displacement of the fluid and cupula in the narrow semicircular canals. Because of the great flexibility of the basilar membrane, the range of sound frequencies to which the hair cells in the cochlea are sensitive varies from 20 to 20,000 Hz.

The effective stimulus to the sensory cells in the labyrinth is the relative displacement of the cilia produced by the application of mechanical force to the cilia's surroundings.

THE EIGHTH NERVE

The eighth nerve, a combination of the **auditory** and **vestibular nerves**, enters the posterior cranial fossa through the internal auditory canal (Fig. 13). The auditory nerve, consisting of approxi-

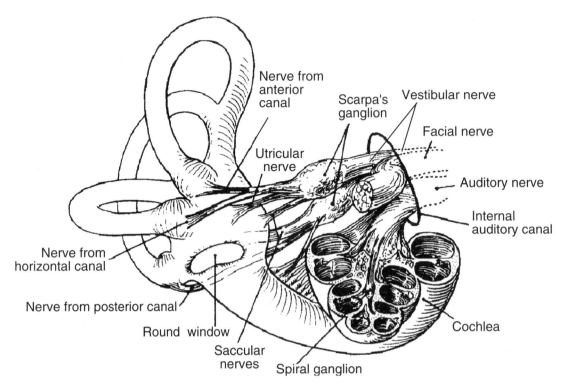

FIGURE 13 Innervation of the labyrinth.

mately 30,000 fibers, occupies the anterior inferior part of the internal auditory canal, and the vestibular nerve, containing approximately 20,000 fibers, occupies the posterior half. The facial nerve is located in the remaining anterior superior quadrant.

The afferent bipolar ganglion cells of the vestibular nerve (Scarpa's ganglion) are arranged in two cell masses in a vertical column, the superior group forming the superior division of the vestibular nerve and the inferior group forming the inferior division. The superior division innervates the cristae of the anterior and horizontal canals, the macule of the utricle, and the anterior superior part of the macule of the saccule. The inferior division innervates the crista of the posterior canal and the main portion of the saccule. The bipolar cochlear neurons are located in the spiral ganglion of the cochlea. As with the vestibular nerve, the orderly spatial arrangement of the cochlear neurons within the spiral ganglion is maintained in the nerve trunk. The nerve fibers from the basal turn of the cochlea are located in the peripheral and inferior portions of the nerve trunk, and the apical fibers are in the central region.

References

1. Gray O: A brief survey of the phylogenesis of the labyrinth. J Laryngol Otol 69:151, 1955.
2. Wersall DJ, and Bagger-Sjoback D: Morphology of the vestibular sense organs. In Kornhuber HH (ed): Handbook of Sensory Physiology, vol. VI, part 2. Springer-Verlag, New York, 1974.

3. Baird LL: Some aspects of the comparative anatomy and evolution of the inner ear in submammalian vertebrates. In Riss W (ed): Brain, Behavior and Evolution. S. Karger, Basel, 1974.

4. Pearson AA: The Development of the Ear: A Manual. American Academy of Ophthalmology and Otolaryngology, Rochester, MN, 1967.

5. Salt AN, and Konishi T: The cochlear fluids: Perilymph and endolymph. In Altschuler RA, Hoffman DW, and Bobbin RP (eds): Neurobiology of Hearing: The Cochlea. Raven Press, New York, 1986.

6. Schuknecht HF: Pathology of the Ear. Lea & Febiger, Philadelphia, 1993.

7. Kimura RS: Animal models of endolymphatic hydrops. Am J Otolaryngol 3:447, 1982.

8. Paparella M: Biochemical Mechanisms of Hearing and Deafness. Charles C Thomas, Springfield, IL, 1970.

9. Schuknecht H, and El Seifi A: Experimental observations on the fluid physiology of the inner ear. Ann Otol Rhinol Laryngol 72:687, 1963.

10. Mazzoni A: Internal auditory artery supply to the petrous bone. Ann Otol Rhinol Laryngol 81:13, 1974.

11. Perlman HB, Kimura RS, and Fernandez C: Experiments on temporary obstruction of the internal auditory artery. Laryngoscope 69: 591, 1959.

12. Flock A, Flock B, and Murray E: Studies on the sensory hair receptor cells in the inner ear. Acta Otolaryngol (Stockh) 83:85, 1977.

13. Shotwell SL, Jocobs R, and Hudspeth AJ: Directional sensitivity of individual vertebrate hair cells to controlled deflection of their hair bundles. In Cohen B (ed): Vestibular and Oculomotor Physiology. Ann N Y Acad Sci 374:1, 1981.

14. Lowenstein OE: Comparative morphology and physiology. In Kornhuber HH (ed): Handbook of Sensory Physiology, vol. VI, part 2. Springer-Verlag, New York, 1974.

15. Hudspeth AJ: The cellular basis of hearing: the biophysics of hair cells. Science 230:745, 1985.

16. Baloh RW, and Honrubia V: Clinical Neurophysiology of the Vestibular System, ed 2. F. A. Davis, Philadelphia, 1990.

17. Fernandez C, and Goldberg JM: Physiology of peripheral neurons innervating otolith organs of the squirrel monkey. I. Response to static tilts and long-duration centrifugal force. J Neurophysiol 39:970, 1976.

18. Fernandez C, and Goldberg JM: Physiology of peripheral neurons innervating otolith organs of the squirrel monkey. II. Directional selectivity and force-response relations. J Neurophysiol 39:985, 1976.

19. Fernandez C, and Goldberg JM: Physiology of peripheral neurons innervating otolith organs of the squirrel monkey. III. Response dynamics. J Neurophysiol 39:996, 1976.

20. Fernandez C, Goldberg JM, and Baird RA: The vestibular nerve of the chinchilla. III. Peripheral innervation patterns of the utricular macula. J Neurophysiol 63:767, 1990.

21. Blanks RHI, Curthoys IS, and Markham CH: Planar relationships of the semicircular canals in man. Acta Otolaryngol (Stockh) 80:185, 1975.

22. Highstein SM: How does the vestibular part of the inner ear work? In Baloh RW, and Halmagyi GM (eds): Disorders of the Vestibular System. Oxford University Press, New York, 1996.

23. Goldberg J, and Fernandez C: Physiology of peripheral neurons innervating semicircular canals of the squirrel monkey. I. Resting discharge and response to constant angular accelerations. J Neurophysiol 34:635, 1971.

24. Fernandez C, and Goldberg J: Physiology of peripheral neurons innervating semicircular canals of the squirrel monkey. II. Response to sinusoidal stimulation and dynamics of peripheral system. J Neurophysiol 34:661, 1971.

25. Goldberg J, and Fernandez C: Physiology of peripheral neurons innervating semicircular canals of the squirrel monkey. III. Variations among units in their discharge properties. J Neurophysiol 34:676, 1971.

26. Santi PA, and Mancicni P: Cochlear anatomy and central auditory pathways. In Cummings CW, et al (eds): Otolaryngology — Head and Neck Surgery, vol. 4. Mosby Year Book, St. Louis, 1993.

27. Gelfand SA: Hearing: an introduction to psychological and physiological acoustics. Marcel Dekker, New York, 1990.

28. Gulick WL, Gescheider GA, and Frisina RD: Hearing: Physiological Acoustics, Neural Coding and Psychoacoustics. Oxford University Press, New York, 1989.

29. Sutton S, and Schuknecht H: Regional hearing loss from induced cochlear injuries in experimental animals. Ann Otol Rhinol Laryngol 63:727, 1954.

3

The Central Vestibular System

THE VESTIBULAR NUCLEI

The central processes of the primary afferent vestibular neurons divide into an ascending and descending branch after entering the brain stem at the inner aspect of the restiform body (Fig. 14).[1] The ascending branch ends either in the rostral end of the vestibular nuclei or in the cerebellum, and the descending branch ends in the caudal vestibular nuclei. The vestibular nuclei consist of a group of neurons located on the floor of the fourth ventricle, bounded laterally by the restiform body, ventrally by the nucleus and spinal tract of the trigeminal nerve, and medially by the pontine reticular formation.[2] Four distinct anatomic groups of neurons have traditionally been identified: the **medial**, **lateral**, **superior**, and **inferior nuclei** (see Fig. 14). Although there is considerable overlap, most fibers originating from the utricle and the saccule end in the lateral and inferior nuclei, and most fibers originating from the semicircular canals terminate in the superior

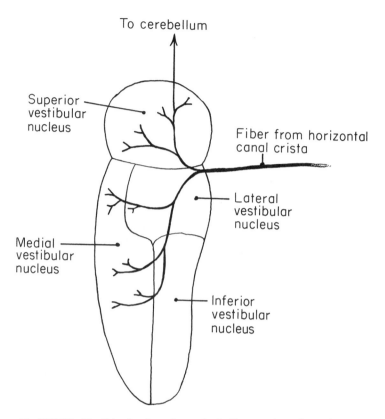

FIGURE 14 Distribution of a typical afferent nerve from the horizontal semicircular canal within the vestibular nuclei. (Adapted from Gacek, R: The course and central termination of first order neurons supplying vestibular end organs in the cat. Acta Otolaryngol Suppl 254, 1969.)

and medial nuclei. The vestibular nuclei receive signals from the cerebellum, the cervical spinal cord, and the nearby reticular formation in addition to those from the vestibular afferent projections. There are also large numbers of interconnecting commissural fibers between the vestibular nuclei on both sides. Based on the combined afferent and efferent fiber connections, the lateral and inferior vestibular nuclei are important relay stations for control of vestibulospinal reflexes, whereas the superior and medial nuclei are critical stations for control of the vestibulo-ocular reflexes.

The lateral and inferior vestibular nuclei are important relay stations for the control of vestibulospinal reflexes, and the superior and medial nuclei are critical for control of the vestibulo-ocular reflexes.

VESTIBULO-OCULAR REFLEXES

General Organization

Connections between the vestibular nuclei and the oculomotor neurons run in two separate pathways: One is a direct pathway from secondary vestibular neurons to oculomotor neurons, and the other is an indirect pathway relayed through the reticular substance of the brain stem.[3] Many of the direct connections from the vestibular nuclei to the oculomotor nuclei are part of a large fiber bundle, the **medial longitudinal fasciculus (MLF)**, lying along the floor of the fourth ventricle. This fiber bundle extends from the cervical cord to the reticular substance of the midbrain and thalamus, providing an interconnecting pathway between the vestibular and the abducens nuclei in the middle brain stem and the oculomotor complex in the rostral brain stem. The indirect pathway between the vestibular and oculomotor nuclei is multisynaptic, involving both short and long axonal interconnections within the reticular substance.

Precise vestibulo-ocular control requires the combination of activity in both pathways. Vestibulo-ocular reflexes are reduced, but not abolished, by sectioning the axons in the MLF or by lesions in the pontine reticular formation.[4] The direct and indirect pathways complement each other; the direct pathways provide a quick communication channel, and the indirect pathways act as a modulator. By reverberating (feedback) circuits, the indirect pathway maintains a level of spontaneous activity, or tonus, and integrates information from several neural centers (the so-called **velocity storage** system).[5] It creates the necessary delays for summation of signals from the visual, proprioceptive, and vestibular systems to produce accurate compensatory eye movements. It acts, therefore, as a fine tuner of vestibular-induced eye movements.

The direct vestibulo-ocular pathways provide a quick communication channel, and the indirect pathways act as a modulator.

Canal-Ocular Connections

The afferent nerves from each semicircular canal are connected to the motoneurons of the eye muscles in such a way that stimulation of the nerve from a given canal results in eye movement in the plane of that canal.[3] For example, stimulation of the ampullary nerve from the left posterior canal causes excitation of the left superior oblique and right inferior rectus muscles while inhibiting the left inferior oblique and right superior rectus. An oblique downward movement in the plane of the left posterior canal is the end result. As we will see later, these connections explain the torsional vertical nystagmus seen with benign positional vertigo.

The afferent nerves from each semicircular canal are connected to the motor neurons of the eye muscles in such a way that stimulation of the nerve from a given canal results in eye movements in the plane of that canal.

The direct pathways from the horizontal canals to the horizontal extraocular muscles (Fig. 15) deserve particular attention, since the horizontal vestibulo-ocular reflex is the focus of many clinical vestibular tests. The secondary vestibular neurons lie in the medial and lateral vestibular nucleus.[6] The more medial group of excitatory neurons projects to the contralateral abducens nucleus, while the more laterally located excitatory neurons (in the medial part of the lateral nucleus) project to ipsilateral medial rectus motoneurons via the **ascending tract of Deiters (ATD)**. The ipsilateral medial rectus neurons also receive a strong excitatory input via the MLF from interneurons in the contralateral abducens nucleus. These interneurons are excited by the same secondary vestibular neurons that excite the abducens motor neurons.[7] The relative contributions to the horizontal vestibulo-ocular reflex of

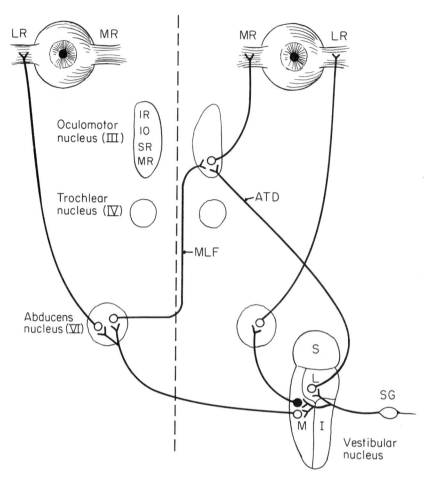

FIGURE 15 Direct pathways of the horizontal semicircular canal-ocular reflex. The darkened cell body indicates an inhibitory secondary vestibular neuron. SG = Scarpa's ganglion, S = superior nucleus, L = lateral nucleus, M = medial nucleus, I = inferior nucleus, MLF = medial longitudinal fasciculus, ATD = ascending tract of Deiters, IR = inferior rectus, IO = inferior oblique, SR = superior rectus, MR = medial rectus, LR = lateral rectus.

the ATD and MLF excitatory pathways are not entirely clear, but the MLF pathway seems more important; the eyes cannot adduct past the midline if the MLF is sectioned.[8] Inhibitory secondary neurons in the rostral part of the medial vestibular nucleus run directly to the ipsilateral abducens nucleus. Contralateral medial rectus motoneurons apparently do not receive disynaptic inhibition from the horizontal semicircular canals.[6,7]

In addition to the direct and indirect connections between secondary vestibular neurons and oculomotor neurons, commissural connections between the two vestibular nuclei play an important role in controlling the vestibulo-ocular reflex.[9] Through inhibitory interneurons, secondary vestibular neurons on one side inhibit their counterparts on the opposite side. The commissural connections are particularly important after unilateral loss of vestibular function since they provide a mechanism for a single labyrinth to control the vestibular nuclei on both sides, thus maintaining a

The commissural connections between the vestibular nuclei are particularly important after unilateral loss of vestibular function, because they enable a single labyrinth to control the vestibular nuclei on both sides.

functional vestibulo-ocular reflex (see Vestibular Rehabilitation in Chapter 11).

Because physiological stimuli activate both labyrinths, the horizontal vestibulo-ocular reflex is controlled by a four-way, push-pull mechanism.[4] For example, physiological stimulation of the crista of the right horizontal semicircular canal excites the left lateral rectus and the right medial rectus and inhibits the right lateral rectus. Because of the symmetry between the labyrinths, the same receptor in the other ear simultaneously diminishes its afferent output, thereby disfacilitating the left medial rectus and right lateral rectus and disinhibiting the left lateral rectus. The end result is contraction of the left lateral and right medial rectus muscles and relaxation of the left medial and right lateral rectus muscles.

Nystagmus

If a subject is rotated back and forth in the dark in the plane of the horizontal semicircular canals, compensatory eye movements are induced, with eye velocity approximately equal and opposite to the head velocity.[3,4] If the angle of rotation is large, such that it cannot be compensated for by motion of the eye in the orbit, the slow compensatory vestibular-induced eye deviation is interrupted by quick movements in the opposite direction. This combination of rhythmic slow and fast eye movements is called **nystagmus**. Because of the fast components, the trajectory of the eye motion during the slow components effectively compensates for head rotation as if the eye had unlimited freedom of motion. Without the fast components, the eyes would become pinned in an extreme orbital position and the vestibulo-ocular reflex would cease functioning.

Spontaneous nystagmus occurs after lesions of the labyrinth, the vestibular nerve and the central vestibulo-ocular neurons, and interconnecting pathways.[4] The key ingredient for the production of spontaneous nystagmus is an imbalance of tonic signals within the vestibulo-ocular pathways. Damage to one labyrinth or one vestibular nerve results in spontaneous nystagmus, with the slow phase directed toward the side of the lesion; the tonic input from the intact side is no longer balanced by input from the damaged side. This spontaneous nystagmus is indistinguishable from nystagmus produced by physiological stimulation of the opposite normal vestibular nerve (Fig. 16). The direction of spontaneous nystagmus associated with lesions in the brain stem is less predictable, depending on the location and extent of the lesion. Central spontaneous nystagmus can be purely vertical or torsional, since tonic signals to the oblique and vertical rectus muscles run in separate pathways from those of the vestibular nuclei.

Groups of neurons in the **paramedian pontine reticular formation (PPRF)** immediately adjacent to the abducens nuclei fire in short bursts of activity just before the onset of horizontal fast components.[3,10] Numerous pathways interconnect neurons in the vestibular nuclei with neurons in this region of the PPRF, and the

The key ingredient for spontaneous nystagmus is an imbalance of tonic signals within the vestibulo-ocular pathways.

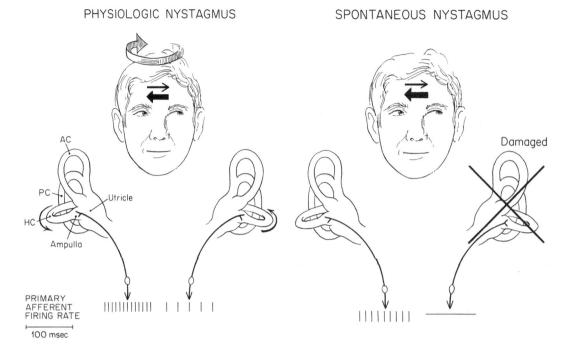

PHYSIOLOGIC NYSTAGMUS   SPONTANEOUS NYSTAGMUS

AC

PC   Utricle

HC

Ampulla

Damaged

PRIMARY
AFFERENT
FIRING RATE

100 msec

FIGURE 16   Primary afferent nerve activity associated with rotation-induced physiological nystagmus and spontaneous nystagmus resulting from a lesion of one labyrinth. The thin straight arrows indicate the direction of slow components; the thick straight arrows indicate the direction of fast components; curved arrows show the direction of endolymph flow in the horizontal semicircular canals. AC = anterior canal, PC = posterior canal, HC = horizontal canal.

Unilateral lesions of the paramedian pontine reticular formation (PPRF) impair ipsilateral rapid eye movements, and the eyes deviate to the contralateral side. Stimuli that normally would produce nystagmus with ipsilateral fast components simply cause strong tonic contralateral deviation.

latter project directly to oculomotor neurons and interneurons in the abducens nucleus. Apparently neurons in the PPRF monitor vestibulo-ocular signals and intermittently fire in bursts to produce corrective fast components based on certain features of the signal, particularly the eye position in the orbit. During angular rotation, the fast components of the initial beats of nystagmus attain a larger amplitude than the preceding slow components, and the eyes deviate in the direction of the fast component.[4] The apparent advantage of this strategy is that the eyes are ready to focus on newly arriving targets in the field of rotation, and fixation can be maintained during the subsequent slow component. Unilateral lesions of the PPRF impair ipsilateral rapid eye movements, and the eyes deviate to the contralateral side of the orbit.[11] Stimuli that normally would produce nystagmus with ipsilateral fast components simply cause a strong tonic contralateral deviation of the eyes.

Otolith-Ocular Connections

The pathways from the macules to the extraocular muscles are less clearly defined than those from the semicircular canals.[6] Because of the varied orientation of hair cells within the macules (see Fig. 9), simultaneous stimulation of all the nerve fibers coming from a macule produces a nonphysiological excitation, and the induced eye movements fail to represent the naturally occurring ones. Selective stimulation of different parts of the utricle and saccule results in mostly vertical and vertical-rotatory eye movements.[12] As one would expect, stimulation on each side of the striola produces oppositely directed rotatory and vertical components.

To simplify the discussion of the otolith-ocular reflexes, it is helpful to think of the otolith organs (the utricular and saccular macules combined) as a unitary sensor capable of resolving all the linear forces acting on the head into a single vector force. This "unitary" three-dimensional otolith receptor is positioned at the center of the head with the x- and z-axes orthogonal to the earth's vertical axis and the y-axis parallel to it. The receptor computes the angle (θ) between the resultant vector force and the earth's vertical axis and sends this information to the brain, where a compensatory eye deviation is generated with the goal of maintaining the eyes in a normal position relative to the earth's vertical axis (Fig. 17). The perfect otolith-ocular reflex would be one that rotates the eyes at an angle equal and opposite to θ. In the case of head tilt in the x-y plane, as illustrated in Figure 17B, the efficiency or gain of the reflex can be represented by the relationship between the angle of eye deviation to the angle of head tilt θ (gain = α/θ).

With this concept in mind, it is interesting to compare the eye movements produced by head tilt (Fig. 17B) with those produced by linear displacement of the head (Fig. 17C). During static head tilt θ is equal to the angle of tilt and the resulting ocular rotation α compensates for the tilt, maintaining the eyes in the horizontal plane. The otolith signal also provides the brain with an aware-

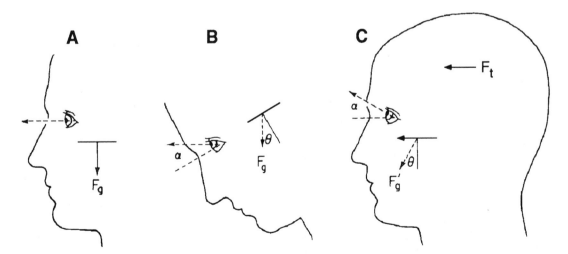

FIGURE 17   Otolith-ocular responses. (A) The force of gravity (F_g) is orthogonal to the line of sight. Compensatory eye movements are induced by static head tilt (B) and by linear acceleration (F_t) tangential to the "unitary" otolith receptor (C). α = the angle of eye rotation and θ = the angle between the resultant force of gravity (F_g') and a line orthogonal to the receptor. (From Baloh, RW and Honrubia, V: *Clinical Neurophysiology of the Vestibular System,* ed. 2. F.A. Davis, Philadelphia, 1990, p 59, with permission.)

ness of the true vertical (the direction of the gravitational vector F_g). The situation is different when linear acceleration is applied parallel to the x-axis (Fig. 17C). If a linear force F_t is chosen that is exactly equal to the force produced by static head tilt in Figure 17B, the eye rotation α will be the same as that associated with the head tilt. This poses an interesting problem for the brain—how to distinguish between forces associated with head tilt and those associated with linear acceleration. This problem is usually not difficult, since most linear accelerations associated with natural head movements are brief, high-frequency displacements rather than low-frequency, constant acceleration of gravity. If a subject is exposed to a constant linear acceleration parallel to the x-axis, as shown in Figure 17C, however, the subject will erroneously interpret the direction of the force of gravity as that of the earth vertical and will have an illusion of tilt determined by the angle θ.

Interaction with Visual and Neck Proprioceptive Signals

Visual, proprioceptive, and vestibular signals interact synergistically to stabilize gaze during most natural head movements.[4] The effect is better ocular stability than would be possible if each system worked alone. Occasionally these signals conflict, and one must override the others to maintain gaze stability. For example, when the head and visual target are moving at the same velocity, the vestibulo-ocular and nuchal-ocular reflexes are suppressed and gaze is maintained on the target.

Secondary vestibular neurons receive afferent visual and proprioceptive signals in addition to primary vestibular signals (Fig. 18).[13] The visual and proprioceptive signals are organized such that movement of the visual surround in one direction excites and inhibits the same neurons that are excited and inhibited by movement of the head and neck in the opposite direction. The vestibular nucleus is therefore not simply a relay station for vestibular reflexes but rather an important sensorimotor interaction center.

The vestibular nucleus is an important sensorimotor interaction center, not simply a relay station for vestibular reflexes.

Visual signals reach the vestibular nuclei by at least two different pathways: a cortical pathway with relay stations in the geniculate ganglion and parieto-occipital cortex and a subcortical pathway with relay stations in the pretectum.[13,14] Details on the exact pathways to the vestibular nuclei from these visual centers are poorly understood, but the cerebellum (particularly the flocculonodular lobes) appears to be a critical relay station for both pathways. Monkeys who have undergone flocculectomy and humans with midline cerebellar lesions are unable to inhibit vestibular signals with visual signals.[15,16] Floccular Purkinje cells receive primary vestibular afferent signals and visual signals and in turn send out impulses to second-order neurons of the vestibulo-ocular reflex arc. Apparently the flocculus "compares" visual and vestibular signals, and if the signals conflict with each other, the

Humans with midline cerebellar lesions are unable to inhibit vestibular signals with visual signals.

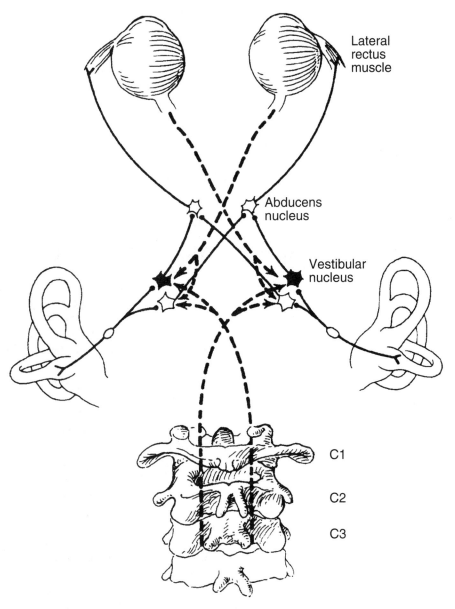

FIGURE 18 Visual-nuchal-vestibular interaction at secondary vestibular neurons within the horizontal semicircular canal ocular reflex. Black = inhibitory neuron; white = excitatory neuron.

characteristics of the vestibular response are changed at the level of the vestibular nucleus.[17]

Neck proprioceptive signals originate from receptors deep in the ligaments and joints of the upper cervical vertebrae (C1–C3) and interact with afferent vestibular signals at the vestibular nucleus (see Fig. 18).[4,18] Stimulation of the neck joint receptors activates neurons in the contralateral vestibular nucleus that are part of the canal-ocular pathways. Turning the head to the right stretches the joint ligaments and thereby activates receptors in the left side of the neck. This activity excites neurons in the right vestibular nucleus, which in turn excites neurons in the left abducens nucleus and right oculomotor nucleus. Inhibitory interneurons in the vestibular nuclei are also activated by afferent nerve signals from the neck to maintain the necessary balance between excitation of agonist muscles and inhibition of antagonist muscles. Unilateral interruption of cervical proprioceptive signals by either root section or local anesthetic block produces nystagmus in animals and vertigo in human subjects.[19] Compared with the labyrinthine input to the vestibular nuclei, however, cervical input is minor, and its interruption results in relatively mild functional loss for which there is rapid compensation.

> *Unilateral interruption of cervical proprioceptive signals produces vertigo in human subjects. Compared with the labyrinthine input to the vestibular nuclei, however, cervical input is minor and its interruption causes relatively mild functional loss for which there is rapid compensation.*

VESTIBULOSPINAL REFLEXES

Secondary vestibular neurons influence spinal anterior horn cell activity by means of three major pathways: (1) the lateral vestibulospinal tract, (2) the medial vestibulospinal tract, and (3) the reticulospinal tract.[2,20] The first two arise directly from neurons in the vestibular nuclei (Fig. 19); the third arises from neurons in the reticular formation that are influenced by vestibular stimulation (as well as several other kinds of input). The cerebellum is highly interrelated with each of these pathways.

Lateral Vestibulospinal Tract

Most fibers in the lateral vestibulospinal tract originate from neurons in the lateral vestibular nucleus.[2] A somatotropic pattern of projections originates in this nucleus such that neurons in the rostroventral region supply the cervical cord, while neurons in the dorsocaudal region innervate the lumbosacral cord. Neurons in the intermediate region supply the thoracic cord. Although the lateral vestibulospinal tract is largely uncrossed, a small component of the pathway reaches the contralateral gray matter via the spinal ventral gray commissure. Electric stimulation in the lateral nucleus produces monosynaptic excitation of ipsilateral extensor motoneurons and disynaptic inhibition of contralateral flexor motoneurons.

Medial Vestibulospinal Tract

The fibers of the medial vestibulospinal tract originate from neurons in the medial vestibular nucleus and enter the spinal cord in the descending MLF.[2] The fibers travel in the ventral funicle as far as the midthoracic level. Most end on interneurons in the cervical cord. No monosynaptic connections appear to exist between the medial vestibulospinal tract and the cervical anterior horn cells.

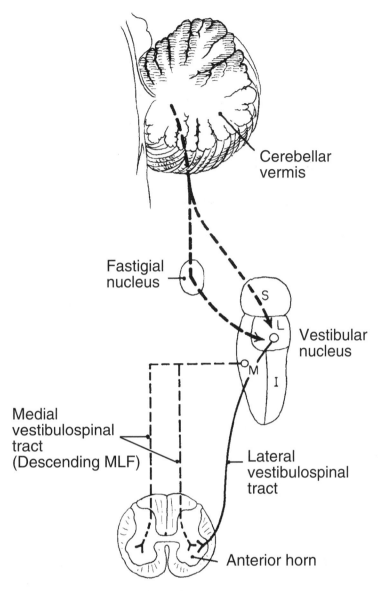

Cerebellar
vermis

Fastigial
nucleus

S

L

Vestibular
nucleus

M

I

Medial
vestibulospinal
tract
(Descending MLF)

Lateral
vestibulospinal
tract

Anterior horn

FIGURE 19 Vestibulospinal pathways. Thin dashed lines represent multisynaptic connections of the medial vestibulospinal tract; heavy dashed lines represent the strong influence of the cerebellar vermis on secondary vestibular neurons, giving rise to the lateral vestibulospinal tract.

Reticulospinal Tract

The reticulospinal tract originates from neurons in the bulbar reticular formation.[21] The nuclei reticularis gigantocellularis and pontis caudalis provide most of the long fibers passing into the spinal cord, although most neurons in the caudal reticular formation also contribute fibers. Only a few primary vestibular fibers end in the reticular formation; the main vestibular influence on reticulospinal outflow is mediated by way of the secondary vestibular neurons. A pattern exists within the vestibuloreticular projections such that each nucleus projects to a different area of the reticular formation, but no detailed somatotopic organization has been identified. Both crossed and uncrossed fibers traverse the length of the spinal cord. Stimulation of the pontomedullary reticular formation in the regions where the long descending spinal projections originate results in inhibition of both extensor and flexor motoneurons throughout the spinal cord.

Cerebellar-Vestibular Pathways

The midline or "spinal" cerebellum provides a major source of input to neurons whose axons form the lateral vestibulospinal and reticulospinal tracts.[20] A somatotopic organization of projections to the lateral nucleus occurs in both the vermian cortex and the fastigial nuclei. Direct projections connect the vermian cortex to the lateral vestibular nucleus, and indirect projections pass through the fastigial nuclei (see Fig. 19). The caudal part of the fastigial nucleus gives rise to a bundle of fibers that crosses the midline (Russell's hook bundle), curving around the brachium conjunctivum before running to the contralateral lateral vestibular nucleus and dorsolateral reticular formation. In addition, direct ipsilateral outflow passes from the fastigial nucleus to areas of the reticular formation that send long fibers to the spinal cord in the reticulospinal tract. The cerebellar reticular pathways do not exhibit somatotopic organization.

The cerebellar vermis and fastigial nuclei receive input from secondary vestibular neurons, the spinal cord, and the pontomedullary reticular formation. The result is a close-knit vestibular-reticular-cerebellar functional unit for the maintenance of equilibrium and locomotion.

Vestibular Influence on Posture and Equilibrium

The anterior horn cells of the antigravity muscles are under the combined excitatory and inhibitory influence of multiple supraspinal neural centers.

The anterior horn cells of the antigravity muscles (extensors of the neck, trunk, and extremities) are under the combined excitatory and inhibitory influence of multiple supraspinal neural centers.[4] At least in the cat, one finds two main facilitatory centers (the lateral vestibular nucleus and the rostral reticular formation) and four inhibitory centers (the pericruciate cortex, the basal ganglia, the cerebellum, and the caudal reticular formation). The balance of input from these different centers determines the degree of tone in the antigravity muscles. If one removes the inhibitory influence of the frontal cortex and basal ganglia by sectioning the animal's midbrain, a characteristic state of contraction in the antigravity muscles results, called "decerebrate rigidity." The extensor muscles increase their resistance to lengthening, and the deep tendon reflexes become hyperactive. The vestibular system contributes largely to this increased extensor tone, which markedly decreases after bilateral destruction of the labyrinths. Destruction of one labyrinth or lateral vestibular nucleus causes an ipsilateral decrease in tone, indicating that the main excitatory input to the anterior horn cells arrives from the ipsilateral lateral vestibulospinal tract.

In a decerebrate animal with normal labyrinths, the intensity of the extensor tone can be modulated in a specific way by changing the position of the head in space. For example, if the head of the upright animal is tilted upward, extensor tone in the forelegs increases; downward tilting of the head causes decreased extensor tone and flexion of the forelegs. Lateral tilt produces extension of the extremities on the opposite side. These tonic labyrinthine reflexes, mediated by way of the otoliths, seldom occur in intact animals or human subjects because of the inhibitory influence of the higher cortical and subcortical centers. They can be demonstrated in premature infants, however, and in adults with lesions releasing the brain stem from the higher neural centers.

VESTIBULOCORTICAL PROJECTIONS

Several clinical observations support the existence of a specific vestibular sensation. Patients with either congenital or acquired lack of vestibular function do not experience a turning sensation when rotated in the dark, eliminating visual and tactile cues. Patients with complete spinal transections in the cervical region, on the other hand, perceive acceleration of the head and body normally. The sensation of movement is not dependent on vision or associated nystagmus; blind subjects and patients with complete oculomotor paralysis experience a spinning sensation comparable to that of normal subjects when their vestibular end organs are stimulated. Epileptic discharges from many different areas of the cortex can be associated with a subjective illusion of movement (usually spinning), implying a cerebrocortical representation for vestibular sensation.

The ascending vestibulocortical system includes at least three synaptic stations: the vestibular nuclei, the thalamus, and the cerebral cortex.[22] Vestibulothalamic projections originate from neurons in the superior and lateral vestibular nuclei. At least two thalamic regions receive projections from these secondary vestibular neurons.[21] A large anterior vestibulothalamic projection runs ventrally in the brain stem, passing lateral to the red nucleus and dorsal to the subthalamic nucleus, to terminate in the main sensory nucleus of the thalamus (nucleus ventralis posterior lateralis pars oralis) (Fig. 20). A smaller posterior vestibulothalamic projection runs in the lateral lemniscus along with the auditory projections and ends predominantly near the medial geniculate. Nearly all vestibulothalamic projections run outside the MLF. Two separate thalamocortical projection areas have been identified in the monkey: one near the central sulcus close to the motor cortex and the other at the lower end of the intraparietal sulcus,

Epileptic discharges from many different areas of the cortex can be associated with the subjective illusion of movement (usually spinning), implying a cerebrocortical representation of vestibular sensation.

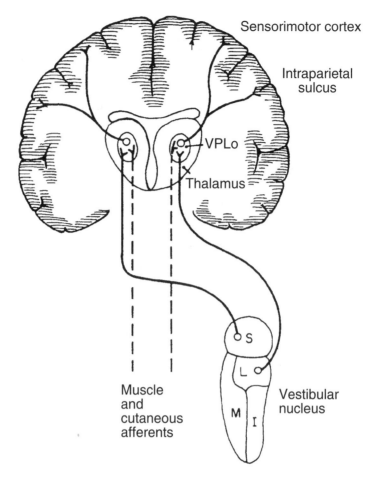

FIGURE 20   Vestibulothalamocortical projections. S = superior nucleus, L = lateral nucleus, M = medial nucleus, I = inferior nucleus, VPLo = nucleus ventralis posterior lateralis pars oralis.

The vestibulothalamocortical projections appear to integrate vestibular, proprioceptive, and visual signals to provide one with a "conscious awareness" of body orientation.

next to the face area of the postcentral gyrus. In humans, electrical stimulation of the superior sylvian gyrus and the region of the inferior intraparietal sulcus produces a subjective sensation of rotation or body displacement.[23]

The vestibulocortical pathway via the thalamus is concerned with the control of body position and orientation in space. Thalamic and cortical units that receive vestibular signals are also activated by proprioception and visual stimuli (as shown in Fig. 20). Most units respond in a similar way to rotation in the dark or to moving visual fields, indicating that they play a role in relaying information about self-motion. From a functional point of view, the vestibulothalamocortical projections appear to integrate vestibular, proprioceptive, and visual signals to provide one with a "conscious awareness" of body orientation. Beginning at the vestibular nuclei, a stepwise integration of body-orienting signals occurs, reaching its maximum at the level of the cortex.

THE VESTIBULAR EFFERENT SYSTEM

Peripheral vestibular efferent fibers originate from approximately 300 neurons located bilaterally ventromedial to the ventral portion of the lateral vestibular nucleus.[24] These fibers accompany the cochlear efferent fibers (the so-called **olivocochlear bundle**) in the vestibular nerve trunk as far as the saccular ganglion, at which point the two efferent systems diverge almost at right angles to each other. Vestibular efferent fibers join each division of the vestibular nerve and run to each macule and crista. Here they end as vesiculated boutons containing many small homogeneous vesicles (see Fig. 8). One efferent fiber gives off numerous boutons that will synapse either directly on hair cells or onto their afferent nerve endings. Pharmacologically the efferent fibers and their terminals contain a high concentration of the enzyme acetylcholinesterase, indicating that acetylcholine is probably the peripheral synaptic transmitter.

The functional significance of the vestibular efferent system in humans is yet to be determined. Studies in the cat and frog suggest a tonic inhibitory influence of the efferent system on spontaneous afferent activity.[25] In the monkey, however, electrical excitation of the central efferent pathways (ipsilateral or contralateral) increases the afferent background activity monitored in Scarpa's ganglion.[26] Thus, there may be species differences in the role of the vestibular efferent system, or the system may have a dual influence, both inhibitory and excitatory, upon the hair cells of the vestibular epithelium.

References

1. Carleton SC, and Carpenter MB: Distribution of primary vestibular fibers in the brainstem and cerebellum of the monkey. Brain 294:281, 1984.
2. Brodal A: Anatomy of the vestibular nuclei and their connections. In Kornhuber HH (ed): Handbook of Sensory Physiology, vol. VI, part 1. Springer-Verlag, New York, 1974.
3. Markham CH: How does the brain generate horizontal vestibular nystagmus? In Baloh RW, and Halmagyi GH (eds): Disorders of the Vestibular System. Oxford University Press, New York, 1996.
4. Baloh RW, and Honrubia V: Clinical Neurophysiology of the Vestibular System, ed 2. F. A. Davis, Philadelphia, 1990.
5. Cohen B, Henn V, Raphan T, and Dennett D: Velocity storage, nystagmus, and visual vestibular interactions in humans. Ann N Y Acad Sci 374:421, 1981.
6. Buttner-Ennever JA: Vestibular oculomotor organization. In Fuchs AF, and Becker W (eds): The Neural Control of Eye Movements. Elsevier, Amsterdam, 1981.
7. Baker R, and Highstein SM: Vestibular projections to medial rectus subdivision of oculomotor nucleus. J Neurophysiol 41:1629, 1978.
8. Evinger LC, Fuchs AF, and Baker R: Bilateral lesions of the medial longitudinal fasciculus in monkeys: Effects on the horizontal and vertical components of voluntary and vestibular induced eye movements. Exp Brain Res 28:1, 1977.
9. Precht W: The physiology of the vestibular nuclei. In Kornhuber HH (ed): Handbook of Sensory Physiology, vol. VI, part 1. Springer-Verlag, New York, 1974.
10. Henn V, and Cohen B: Activity in motoneurons and brain stem units during eye movements. In Lennerstrand G, and Bach-y-Rita P (eds): Basic

Mechanisms of Ocular Motility and Their Clinical Implications. Pergamon Press, Stockholm, 1975.

11. Henn V, and Buttner V: Disorders of horizontal gaze. In Lennerstrand G, Zee DS, and Keller EL (eds): Functional Basis of Ocular Motility Disorders. Pergamon Press, New York, 1982.

12. Fluur E, and Mellstrom A: The otolith organs and their influence on oculomotor movements. Exp Neurol 30:139, 1971.

13. Waespe W, and Henn V: Gaze stabilization in the primate: The interaction of the vestibulo-ocular reflex, optokinetic nystagmus, and smooth pursuit. Rev Physiol Biochem Pharmacol 106:38, 1987.

14. Hoffman KP: Cortical versus subcortical contributions to the optokinetic reflex in the cat. In Lennerstrand G, Zee DS, and Keller EL (eds): Functional Basis of Ocular Motility Disorders. Pergamon Press, New York, 1982.

15. Zee DS: Ocular motor abnormalities related to lesions in the vestibulo-cerebellum in primate. In Lennerstrand G, Zee DS, and Keller EL (eds): Functional Basis of Ocular Motility Disorders. Pergamon Press, New York, 1982.

16. Baloh RW, Yee RD, Kimm J, and Honrubia V: The vestibulo-ocular reflex in patients with lesions involving the vestibulocerebellum. Exp Neurol 72:141, 1981.

17. Miles FA, and Fuller JG: Visual tracking and the primate flocculus. Science 189:1000, 1975.

18. Hikosaka D, and Maeda M: Cervical effects on abducens motoneurons and their interaction with vestibulo-ocular reflex. Exp Brain Res 18:512, 1973.

19. deJong PTVM, deJong JMBV, Cohen B, and Jongkees LBW: Ataxia and nystagmus induced by injection of local anesthetics in the neck. Ann Neurol 1:240, 1977.

20. Fetter M, and Dichgans J: How do the vestibulo-spinal reflexes work? In Baloh RW, and Halmagyi GM (eds): Disorders of the Vestibular System. Oxford University Press, New York, 1996.

21. Hawrylshyn PA, Rubin AM, Tasker PR, et al: Vestibulothalamic projections in man, a sixth primary sensory pathway. J Neurophysiol 41:394, 1978.

22. Berthoz A: How does the cerebral cortex process and utilize vestibular signals? In Baloh RW, and Halmagyi GM (eds): Disorders of the Vestibular System. Oxford University Press, New York, 1996.

23. Penfield W: Vestibular-sensation and the cerebral cortex. Ann Otol Rhinol Laryngol 66:691, 1957.

24. Gacek R, and Lyon M: The localization of vestibular efferent neurons in the kitten with horseradish peroxidase. Acta Otolaryngol (Stockh) 77:92, 1974.

25. Highstein SM: The efferent control of the organs of balance and equilibrium in the toadfish, Opsanus tau. Ann N Y Acad Sci 656:108, 1992.

26. Goldberg JM, and Fernandez C: Efferent vestibular system in the squirrel monkey: Anatomical localization and influence on afferent activity. J Neurophysiol 43:986, 1980.

4

The Central Auditory System

THE COCHLEAR NUCLEI

At the surface of the brain the **cochlear nucleus** can be seen as a swelling of the cochlear nerve as it enters the dorsolateral brain stem at the junction of the pons and medulla. The nucleus curves upward and medially over the restiform body and is covered superolaterally by the middle cerebellar peduncle. Two major subdivisions are generally recognized: the **dorsal cochlear nucleus** and the **ventral cochlear nucleus**.

Upon entering the brain stem, the primary auditory afferent fibers divide into two branches: an anterior branch that terminates in the anterior part of the ventral cochlear nucleus and a longer posterior branch that further divides, with one branch ending in the posterior part of the ventral cochlear nucleus and the other terminating in the dorsal cochlear nucleus (Fig. 21).[1] Primary cochlear neurons do not bypass the cochlear nucleus or send collaterals beyond it. The orderly spatial arrangement present in the cochlea and the cochlear nerve is maintained in the ventral cochlear nucleus.[2] Axons that originate from cochlear neurons at the basal end of the cochlea terminate in the most medial and rostral areas of the ventral cochlear nucleus, whereas axons originating from neurons in the apex terminate on secondary neurons in the lateral caudal area of the ventral cochlear nucleus.[1]

Neurons in the dorsal cochlear nucleus send their axons into the dorsal trapezoid body, where they cross the midline and ascend in the contralateral lateral lemniscus.[3] The cell bodies of the ventral cochlear nucleus send axons in the ventral trapezoid body

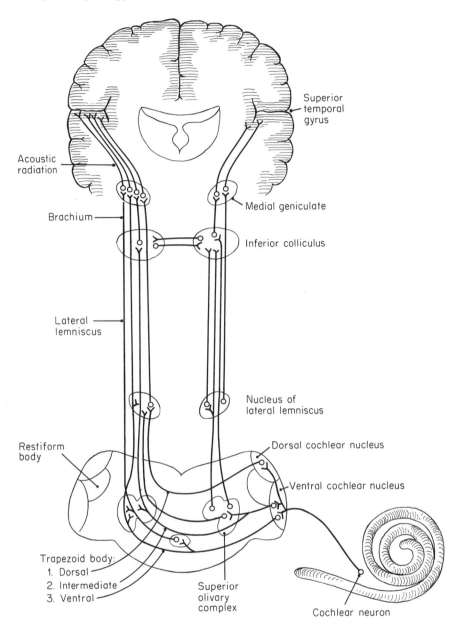

Superior temporal gyrus

Acoustic radiation

Medial geniculate

Brachium

Inferior colliculus

Lateral lemniscus

Nucleus of lateral lemniscus

Dorsal cochlear nucleus

Restiform body

Ventral cochlear nucleus

Trapezoid body:
1. Dorsal
2. Intermediate
3. Ventral

Superior olivary complex

Cochlear neuron

■ **FIGURE 21** Central auditory pathways.

to the ipsilateral and contralateral superior olivary complex. Some of the latter fibers synapse, and others traverse the superior olivary complex and run in the contralateral lateral lemniscus to the inferior colliculus and medial geniculate body.

OTHER PONTINE NUCLEI AND PATHWAYS

Nearly all axons leaving the cochlear nucleus synapse at least once in cell groups between the pontomedullary junction and the midbrain.[3] Three pontine nuclear groups can be identified: the trapezoid nucleus, the superior olivary complex, and the nucleus of the lateral lemniscus (see Fig. 21). The **trapezoid nucleus** receives input from the ventral cochlear nucleus on one side and projects to the lateral lemniscus of the opposite side. The **superior olivary complex** receives input from the ipsilateral and contralateral ventral cochlear nucleus and projects to the nucleus of the lateral lemniscus and the inferior colliculus. The **nucleus of the lateral lemniscus** receives input from the dorsal and the ventral cochlear nuclei, the trapezoid nucleus, and the superior olivary complex and projects to the inferior colliculus and medial geniculate body.

These pontine nuclei function as relay stations for ascending auditory signals and as reflex centers. They represent the first anatomical location where binaural integration of auditory signals occurs consequent to crossing of a roughly equal proportion of afferent auditory fibers. Unilateral hearing loss cannot result from injury to these and the more rostral auditory nuclear groups.

The pontine nuclei are the first anatomical locations where binaural integration of auditory signals occurs, consequent to the crossing of about half of the afferent auditory fibers. Injury to these and the more rostral auditory nuclear groups cannot cause unilateral hearing loss.

THE STAPEDIUS REFLEX

A clinically important auditory reflex is the acoustic or **stapedius reflex** (Fig. 22).[4,5] The stapedius muscle contracts bilaterally in response to sound intensities of 70 to 90 dB above threshold hearing. The reflex activity is maintained for the duration of the stimulus. The stapedius reflex appears to be a protective mechanism to limit the movement of the sound transmitting system in the presence of high-intensity sound. This is not the only function of the reflex, however, since it is also activated by low-intensity sound pressure levels. The stapedius reflex may act in the processing of speech, since patients with stapedius paralysis due to Bell's palsy have impaired ability to discriminate speech.

The reflex arc consists of (1) the hair cells in the organ of Corti, (2) the primary afferent auditory neurons, (3) the ipsilateral secondary neurons in the ventral cochlear nucleus, (4) the bilateral tertiary neurons in the superior olivary nucleus, and (5) the bilateral stapedius motor neurons in the facial nucleus (see Fig. 22). As with the canal-ocular reflex, a parallel multisynaptic pathway from the cochlear nucleus to stapedius motor neurons also exists. If the middle ear structures are intact, loss of the stapedius reflex indicates a lesion of the auditory nerve, the pons, or the facial nerve (see Impedance Audiometry in Chapter 7).

The stapedius reflex may act in processing speech; patients with stapedius paralysis due to Bell's palsy have impaired ability to discriminate speech.

THE INFERIOR COLLICULUS AND MEDIAL GENICULATE BODY

The **inferior colliculi** are two rounded elevations forming the caudal half of the midbrain tectal plate. The main projection of the inferior colliculus is to the ipsilateral medial geniculate body via the brachium of the inferior colliculus (see Fig. 21). The **medial geniculate bodies** are small rounded elevations on the poste-

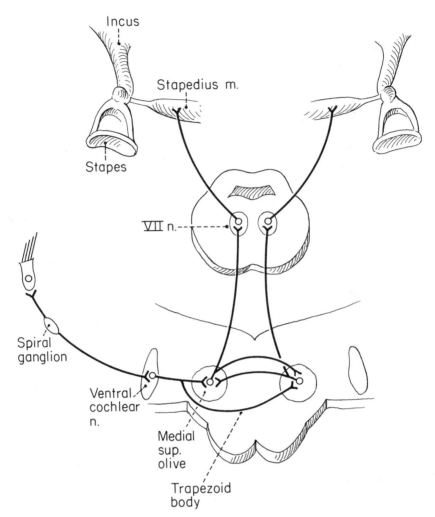

FIGURE 22 The acoustic (stapedius) reflex. Schematic drawing of the direct excitatory connections from the cochlea to the stapedius muscle. (From Baloh, RW: Neurotology. In Joynt, RJ (ed): *Clinical Neurology,* ed 2. J.B. Lippincott, Philadelphia, 1989, with permission.)

rior aspect of each thalamus. No axon of a secondary cochlear neuron reaches the medial geniculate without first synapsing in one of the pontine nuclei or the inferior colliculus, and no ascending neuron bypasses the medial geniculate body.[3] The colliculi have numerous crossover connections, as well as rich connections with the nearby reticular formation, but there are no commissural connections between the medial geniculate bodies.

THE AUDITORY CORTEX

The **auditory cortex** in humans is located in the superior temporal gyrus along the sylvian fissure (see Fig. 21).[2] By Brodmann's classification it corresponds to areas 41, 42, and 22.

Each sensory modality has a primary cortical reception area

surrounded by association areas where integration of primary signals occurs. The primary auditory reception area, Brodmann's area 41, receives its projection from the rostral portion of the pars principalis of the medial geniculate body.[6] An orderly spatial arrangement of tones has been demonstrated in the spiral ganglion of the cochlea, the cochlear nerve trunk, the ventral cochlear nucleus, the superior olivary nucleus, the rostral portions of the medial geniculate body, and the primary auditory cortex. In the primary auditory cortex high frequencies are represented anteriorly and low frequencies posteriorly. Areas 42 and 22, immediately adjacent to the primary auditory cortex, are auditory association areas that receive signals from the primary reception area and project to regions of the occipital, parietal, and insular cortices.

In humans, electrical stimulation close to the margins of the sylvian fissure in the area of the primary auditory cortex produces a sensation of simple sounds, such as a buzzing or ringing. Stimulation away from the fissure, in the association areas, introduces an element of interpretation to the sound, such as a dog barking or a familiar voice.[7] The farther the stimulating electrode moves from the primary reception area, the more complex the interpretation (i.e., the higher the level of integration).

Because of the bilateral representation of hearing at the cortical level, hemispherectomy has no effect on hearing as judged by the pure tone audiogram. Such patients do have impaired discrimination of distorted, interrupted, or accelerated speech, however, particularly when presented to the contralateral ear (see Central Auditory Speech Tests in Chapter 7). Deficits in the production and comprehension of language (aphasia) complicate the clinical analysis of hearing in patients with bilateral lesions of the auditory cortex. In a few cases, bilateral cerebral lesions have produced severe hearing loss in all spheres, not simply an inability to understand spoken language.[8] Recent improvements in brain imaging should lead to better clinical-pathological correlation in such patients.

An orderly spatial arrangement of tones has been demonstrated in the spiral ganglion of the cochlea, the cochlear nerve trunk, the ventral cochlear nucleus, the superior olivary nucleus, the rostral portions of the medial geniculate body, and the primary auditory cortex.

Electrical stimulation in the area of the primary auditory cortex produces a sensation of simple sounds, such as buzzing or ringing, but stimulation in the association areas introduces an element of interpretation to the sound, such as a dog barking or a familiar voice.

THE AUDITORY EFFERENT SYSTEM

A large number of descending neurons parallel the ascending pathways outlined in the preceding sections and link the auditory cortex with the lower auditory centers.[2] The main efferent pathway to the organ of Corti, the **olivocochlear bundle**, originates in the superior olivary complex, with about 75% of fibers coming from the contralateral superior olivary complex and 25% from the ipsilateral side.[9] The fibers from both sides join the vestibular nerve root just beyond the genu of the facial nerve, then send collaterals to the ventral cochlear nucleus as the nerve passes directly beneath it. The auditory efferent fibers emerge from the brain stem in the inferior division of the vestibular nerve and follow this nerve to the cochlea, where they eventually end on afferent nerve endings at the base of the hair cells.

The specific function of the auditory efferent system is yet to

The efferent auditory system may be involved in such behavioral phenomena as attention, frequency discrimination, and detection of signal in noise.

be defined.[10] The widespread branching of each efferent nerve fiber makes it unlikely that they have a localized effect on specific parts of the cochlea. Stimulation of the olivocochlear bundle results in suppression of auditory nerve activity,[11] but sectioning the bundle does not alter behavioral auditory function in the cat.[12] Furthermore, pure tone hearing levels are not affected in patients who have undergone vestibular nerve sectioning for chronic recurrent vertigo. The efferent auditory system may be involved in such behavioral phenomena as attention, frequency discrimination, and detection of signal in noise.

References

1. Sando I: The anatomical interrelationships of the cochlea nerve fibers. Acta Otolaryngol (Stockh) 59:417, 1965.
2. Santi PA, and Mancini P: Cochlear anatomy and central auditory pathways. In Cummings CW, et al (eds): Otolaryngology — Head and Neck Surgery, vol. 4. Mosby Year Book, St. Louis, 1993.
3. Phillips DP: Introduction to Anatomy and Physiology of the Central Auditory Nervous System. Raven Press, New York, 1988.
4. Borg E: On the neuronal organization of the acoustic middle ear reflex. A physiological and anatomical study. Brain Res 49:101, 1973.
5. Zakrisson J, Borg E, and Blom S: The acoustic impedance change as a measure of stapedius muscle activity in man. Acta Otolaryngol (Stockh) 78:157, 1974.
6. Morel A, and Imig TJ: Thalamic projections to fields A, AI, P, VP in the cat auditory cortex. J Comp Neurol 265:119, 1987.
7. Penfield W, and Jasper H: Epilepsy and the Functional Anatomy of the Human Brain. Little, Brown and Co., Boston, 1954.
8. Graham J, Greenwood R, and Lecky B: Cortical deafness. A case report and review of the literature. J Neurol Sci 48:35, 1980.
9. Aschoff A, and Ostwald J: Distribution of cochlear efferents and olivocollicular neurons in the brainstem of rat and guinea pig. Exp Brain Res 71:241, 1988.
10. Abbas PJ: Physiology of the auditory system. In Cummings CW, et al (eds):Otolaryngology — Head and Neck Surgery, vol. 4. Mosby Year Book, St. Louis, 1993.
11. Galambos R: Suppression of auditory nerve activity by stimulation of efferent fibers to cochlea. J Neurophysiol 19:424, 1956.
12. Igarashi M, Alford BR, Nakai Y, et al: Behavioral auditory function after transection of crossed olivo-cochlear bundle in the cat. Acta Otolaryngol (Stockh) 73:455, 1972.

Part II

History and Examination

5

Vestibular Symptoms and Signs

Chapter Outline

SYMPTOMS

As described in preceding chapters, the function of the vestibular system is to transform the forces associated with head acceleration and gravity into a biological signal that the brain can use to develop a subjective awareness of head position in space (orientation) and to produce motor reflexes for postural and ocular stability. Not surprisingly, lesions of the vestibular system commonly result in a sense of disorientation (dizziness), postural and gait imbalance, and visual distortion (oscillopsia).

Lesions of the vestibular system commonly result in disorientation (dizziness), imbalance, and visual distortion (oscillopsia).

Vertigo

Vertigo, an illusion of movement, is specific for vestibular system disease.[1] The most common illusion is that of rotation, although patients occasionally complain of linear displacement or tilt. The afferent nerves from the otoliths and semicircular canals of each labyrinth maintain a balanced tonic rate of firing into the vestibular nuclei. Asymmetry of this baseline activity leads to a sensation of movement. For example, damage to a semicircular canal or its afferent nerve produces a sensation of

Vertigo, an illusion of movement (usually rotation), is specific for vestibular system disease.

angular rotation in the plane of that canal. More commonly, lesions involve all the canals and otoliths of one labyrinth, producing a sensation of rotation in a plane determined by the balance of afferent signals from the other labyrinth (usually near the horizontal, since the vertical canal and otolith signals partially cancel out). If patients with such lesions attempt to fixate on an object, it will appear blurred and seem to be moving in the opposite direction of the slow phase of their spontaneous nystagmus (i.e., away from the side of the lesion). This illusion of movement occurs because the brain lacks eye proprioceptive information and interprets the target displacement on the retina as object movement rather than eye movement. By contrast, if these patients close their eyes, they sense that their body is turning toward the side of the lesion, owing to the imbalance of tonic vestibular signals arriving at the subjective sensation centers of the cortex. An illusion of linear movement alone suggests isolated involvement of an otolith or its central connections.

Although an illusion of movement always indicates an imbalance in the vestibular system (including visual-vestibular and nuchal-vestibular pathways), its absence does not rule out a vestibular lesion. Other descriptions of the sensation associated with vestibular dysfunction include giddiness, swimming in the head, floating, and drunkenness. Symptoms of autonomic dysfunction (e.g., sweating, pallor, nausea, and vomiting) nearly always accompany dizziness caused by vestibular lesions. Occasionally, autonomic symptoms are the only manifestation of such a lesion. Numerous interconnecting pathways between brain stem vestibular and autonomic centers account for this close association of vestibular and autonomic symptoms[2,3] (see Fig. 84).

Vestibular and autonomic symptoms are closely associated.

Imbalance

With acute unilateral vestibular lesions, asymmetry of tonic vestibulospinal activity leads to postural and gait imbalance. The patient tends to fall toward the side of the lesion. This gait unsteadiness is rapidly compensated for, usually lasting less than a week. Patients with a slowly progressive unilateral lesion may not experience any imbalance. Bilateral symmetrical vestibular loss results in a more pronounced and persistent unsteadiness that may be incapacitating in elderly patients,[4] particularly those with other sensory deficits such as peripheral neuropathy and impaired vision (multisensory dizziness).[5] The imbalance due to loss of vestibulospinal or proprioceptive function is typically worse at night, when the patient is less able to use vision to compensate for the vestibular loss. The flowchart in Figure 23 summarizes the logic for distinguishing between vestibular and nonvestibular causes of imbalance.

Imbalance caused by unilateral vestibular lesions is usually transient, but imbalance caused by bilateral vestibular loss is more persistent.

Imbalance

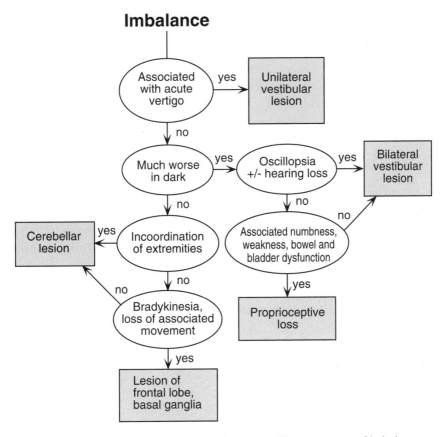

■ **FIGURE 23**   Logic for distinguishing between different causes of imbalance.

Oscillopsia

The optical illusion that stationary objects are moving back and forth or up and down is called **oscillopsia**. Different types of oscillopsia can result from lesions of the vestibulo-ocular pathways. If a patient with an acute unilateral peripheral vestibular lesion attempts to fixate on an object, it will appear blurred and seem to be moving in the opposite direction of the slow phase of the patient's spontaneous nystagmus. This kind of oscillopsia is usually transient, disappearing as the acute vertigo and spontaneous nystagmus disappear. Occasionally, such patients will have persistent head movement–dependent oscillopsia, probably due to inadequate central compensation for the peripheral loss.

Patients with bilateral symmetrical loss of vestibular function develop oscillopsia with any head movement.[6,7] Characteristically, when walking they are unable to fixate on objects because the surroundings are bouncing up and down. To see the faces of passersby, they learn to stop and hold their head still (or say hello to all indiscriminately). When reading, such patients learn to place their hand on their chin to prevent slight movements associ-

Oscillopsia (the illusion that stationary objects are moving back and forth) takes different forms depending on the location of the lesion in the vestibulo-ocular pathways.

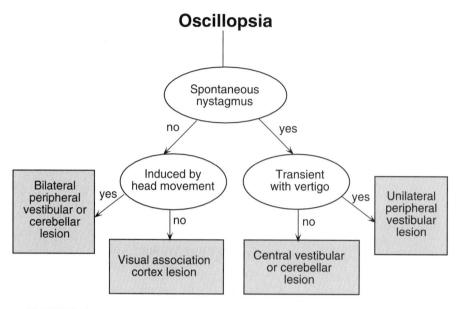

FIGURE 24   Logic for distinguishing between different causes of oscillopsia.

ated with pulsatile cerebral blood flow. Patients with spontaneous nystagmus due to lesions of the central vestibulo-ocular pathways also report oscillopsia, but in this case the oscillopsia is constant and usually associated with other neurologic symptoms. Patients with cerebellar lesions can have oscillopsia at rest because of spontaneous nystagmus or with head movement because they are unable to suppress the vestibulo-ocular reflex with fixation. Rarely, oscillopsia results from a lesion in the parietal occipital cortex. The flowchart in Figure 24 outlines how to distinguish between the different causes of oscillopsia based on the clinical history.

Motion Sickness

Motion sickness is caused by excessive stimulation of the vestibular system, especially when visual signals conflict with the vestibular ones.

Motion sickness refers to the syndrome of dizziness, perspiration, nausea, vomiting, increased salivation, yawning, and generalized malaise caused by excessive stimulation of the vestibular system.[8,9] Although it is usually produced by prolonged stimulation of the labyrinthine end organs, persistent visual stimulation with an optokinetic drum can also produce the syndrome.[10] Both linear and angular head acceleration induce motion sickness in susceptible people if applied for prolonged periods. Combinations of linear and angular acceleration or multiplanar angular accelerations are particularly effective. Rotation about the vertical axis, along with either voluntary or involuntary nodding movements in the sagittal plane, rapidly produce motion sickness in nearly everybody. This movement combines linear and angular acceleration (**Coriolis effect**).

Autonomic symptoms are usually the initial manifestation of motion sickness.[11] Sensitive sweat detectors can identify increased sweating as soon as 5 seconds after onset of motion, and grossly detectable sweating is usually apparent before any noticeable nausea. Increased salivation and frequent swallowing movements occur. Gastric motility is reduced and digestion is impaired. Motion sickness affects the appetite, so that even the sight or smell of food is distressing. In addition, hyperventilation is almost always present, and the resulting hypocapnia leads to changes in blood volume with pooling in the lower parts of the body, predisposing the subject to postural hypotension.

Patients with nonfunctioning labyrinths are immune to motion sickness under all test conditions, even after prolonged exposure to wave motion during a storm at sea, in which all sensory modalities are vigorously stimulated.[11] Some people with normal labyrinths are susceptible to the development of motion sickness, and others are highly resistant. Unfortunately, there is no reliable way to predict who will develop motion sickness. Similarly, although most people eventually adapt to prolonged vestibular stimulation, some never completely adapt (the chronically seasick ocean voyager). Patients with migraine are often very sensitive to motion sickness, and bouts of motion sickness during childhood may be the first symptom of migraine.

An unusual variant of motion sickness is the **mal de debarquement syndrome**.[12] Dizziness begins when the subject returns to stationary conditions after prolonged exposure to motion. Typically, patients report that they feel the persistent rocking sensation of the boat long after returning to dry land. This syndrome can last for months to years after the exposure to motion and occasionally is incapacitating. The cause of the mal de debarquement syndrome is unknown.

Motion sickness seems to result from a visual-vestibular conflict. This theory is supported by the fact that visual influences during body motion have a clear effect on the development of motion sickness.[8] The symptoms are aggravated if one sits in an enclosed cabin on a ship or in the back seat of a moving vehicle. Because the environment is moving with the subject, visual-vestibular conflict occurs. The vestibular system signals movement while the visual system signals a stationary environment. Motion sickness can be alleviated by improving the match between visual and vestibular signals, such as by standing on the deck of a ship and focusing on the distant horizon or on land if possible. When riding in a car, the susceptible person should sit in the front seat to allow ample peripheral vision of the stationary surround. Several drugs that suppress vestibular and autonomic brain stem centers also can relieve many of the symptoms of motion sickness (see Chapter 11).

SIGNS

Postural Instability

Past-Pointing

Past-pointing refers to a reactive deviation of the extremities caused by an imbalance in the vestibular system. The test is performed by having the patient place his or her extended index finger on that of the examiner and with eyes closed raise the extended arm and index finger to a vertical position and attempt to return the index finger to that of the examiner (Fig. 25). Consistent deviation to one side is past-pointing. As with all tests of vestibulospinal function, extralabyrinthine influences should be eliminated as much as possible by having the patient seated with eyes closed and arm and index finger extended throughout the test. Patients with acute peripheral vestibular damage past-point

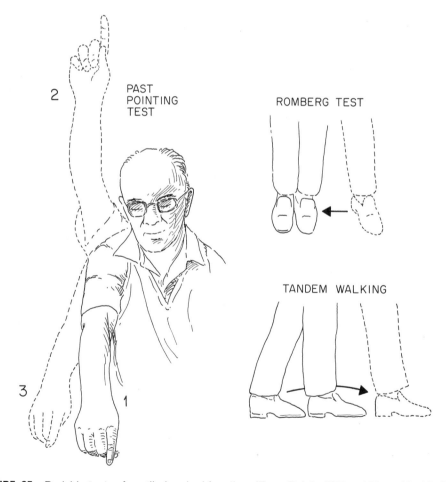

FIGURE 25 Bedside tests of vestibulospinal function. (From Baloh, RW and Honrubia, V: *Clinical Neurophysiology of the Vestibular System*, ed. 2. F.A. Davis, Philadelphia, 1990, p 114, with permission.)

toward the side of loss, but compensation usually corrects the past-pointing and can even produce a drift to the other side. The standard finger-to-nose test will not identify past-pointing since joint and muscle proprioceptive signals permit accurate localization even when vestibular function is lost.

Romberg Test

For the **Romberg test** (see Fig. 25), the patient stands with feet together, arms folded against the chest, and eyes closed. Patients with acute unilateral labyrinthine lesions sway and fall toward the damaged side. Like the past-pointing test, however, the Romberg test is not a good indicator of chronic unilateral vestibular impairment, and sometimes the patient will fall toward the intact side.

With their eyes closed, patients with acute vestibular lesions often will fall during the Romberg test and tandem walking test.

Tandem Walking

When performed with eyes open, **tandem walking**, or heel-to-toe walking (see Fig. 25), is primarily a test of cerebellar function, since vision compensates for chronic vestibular and proprioceptive deficits. Acute vestibular lesions, however, may impair tandem walking even when the eyes are open. Tandem walking with the eyes closed provides a better test of vestibular function, so long as cerebellar and proprioceptive function are intact. As with other tests of vestibulospinal function, however, in patients with chronic lesions the direction of falling is not a reliable indicator of the side of the lesion. So-called stepping or marching tests have the same limitation as the tandem walking test.[13]

Ocular Instability

The Doll's Eye Test

In an alert human, slowly rotating the head back and forth in the horizontal plane induces compensatory horizontal eye movements that are dependent on both the smooth pursuit and the vestibular systems. Rotating the head to the right induces eye movements to the left, and rotating the head to the left induces eye movements to the right. Because of the combined visual and vestibular input, a patient with complete loss of vestibular function and normal pursuit may still have normal compensatory eye movements on this test. The **doll's eye test** is a useful bedside test of vestibular function in a comatose patient, however, since such patients cannot generate pursuit or corrective fast components. In this setting, slow conjugate compensatory eye movements indicate normally functioning vestibulo-ocular pathways (i.e., those illustrated in Fig. 15).

The doll's eye test reveals vestibular function in a comatose patient.

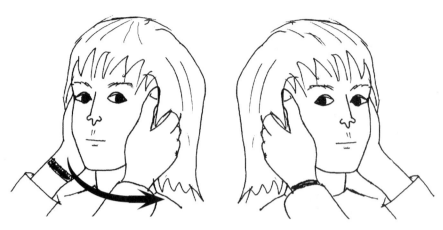

FIGURE 26 The head-thrust test for identifying peripheral vestibular lesions. The head is grasped with both hands and quickly turned first to one side and then the other as the patient attempts to fixate on the examiner's nose. A brief, high-acceleration head thrust should be applied with the eyes beginning about 15° away from primary position in the orbit. The amplitude of head movement should be such that the eyes will end near the primary position of gaze. A corrective saccade (called a catch-up saccade) appears as a sign of an inappropriate compensatory slow phase.

Head-Thrust Test

The head-thrust test identifies unilateral or bilateral loss of vestibular function.

The **head-thrust test** allows one to identify a unilateral or bilateral loss of vestibular function.[14] It is performed by grasping the patient's head and applying brief, small-amplitude, high-acceleration head thrusts, first to one side and then to the other (Fig. 26). The patient fixates on the examiner's nose, and the examiner watches for corrective, "catch-up" saccades, which are a sign of an inappropriate compensatory slow phase. The test is most useful for identifying a unilateral loss of vestibular function because the response to thrusts in one direction can be easily compared with thrusts in the opposite direction. Complete or near-complete bilateral vestibular loss can also be identified, because catch-up saccades will be seen in both directions. The smooth pursuit system is not functional at these high accelerations, so it cannot compensate for the vestibular loss as it does with low-frequency, low-velocity head movements.

Dynamic Visual Acuity Test

Dynamic visual acuity will be poor in a patient with bilateral, symmetrical vestibular damage.

The **dynamic visual acuity test** is performed by having the patient shake the head rapidly back and forth in the horizontal plane at approximately 2 Hz while reading a Snellen visual acuity chart at the standard distance.[15,16] Since the smooth pursuit system functions best below 1 Hz and almost not at all at 2 Hz, this is primarily a test of the horizontal vestibulo-ocular reflex. A drop in acuity of more than one line on the Snellen chart suggests an abnormal vestibulo-ocular reflex, usually due to bilateral, symmetrical damage.

Pathological Nystagmus

Nystagmus is a nonvoluntary, rhythmic oscillation of the eyes that usually has a clearly defined fast and slow component.[1] By convention, the direction of the fast component defines the direction of nystagmus. **Physiological nystagmus** refers to nystagmus that occurs in normal subjects; **pathological nystagmus** implies an underlying abnormality. Physiological nystagmus may be vestibularly induced (rotational or caloric) or visually induced (optokinetic) or may occur on the extremes of lateral gaze (end-point). Pathological nystagmus may be spontaneous (present in the primary position with the patient seated), gaze evoked (induced by change in eye position), or positional (induced by a change in head position). Examination for pathological nystagmus should therefore include a systematic study of changes in fixation, eye position, and head position. In selected patients, pathological nystagmus can be induced after hyperventilation or after head shaking. The features of a pathological nystagmus can be rapidly summarized with a box diagram, as illustrated in Figure 27. The size, shape, and direction of the arrows provide information about the amplitude and direction of the fast component of nystagmus in each eye position.

The direction of nystagmus is the direction of its fast component.

To look for pathological nystagmus, study changes in fixation, eye position, and head position.

Spontaneous Nystagmus

Spontaneous nystagmus results from an imbalance of tonic signals arriving at the oculomotor neurons. Because the vestibular system is the main source of oculomotor tonus, it is the driving force of most types of spontaneous nystagmus. (Tonic signals arising in the pursuit and optokinetic systems may also play a role, particularly with congenital nystagmus.) A vestibular imbalance causes a constant drift of the eyes in one direction, interrupted by fast components in the opposite direction. If the imbalance results from a peripheral vestibular lesion, patients can use their pursuit system to cancel it. If it results from a central vestibular lesion, however, their pursuit system usually cannot suppress it because of the close interrelationship between central vestibular and pursuit pathways. The features that separate peripheral from central varieties of spontaneous nystagmus are summarized in Table 1.

The characteristics of spontaneous nystagmus depend on whether the vestibular lesion is peripheral or central.

A decrease in the baseline flow of action potentials from a single semicircular canal results in nystagmus in the plane of that canal, with a slow conjugate deviation toward the damaged side interrupted by a quick corrective component in the opposite direction (see Fig. 16). Lesions of the peripheral vestibular system (the labyrinth or eighth nerve) typically interrupt tonic afferent signals originating from all of the receptors of one labyrinth, so the resulting nystagmus has combined torsional, horizontal, and vertical components.[17] The horizontal component dominates because the tonic activity from the intact vertical canals partially cancels out. Gaze in the direction of the fast component increases the frequency and amplitude, while gaze in the opposite direction has the

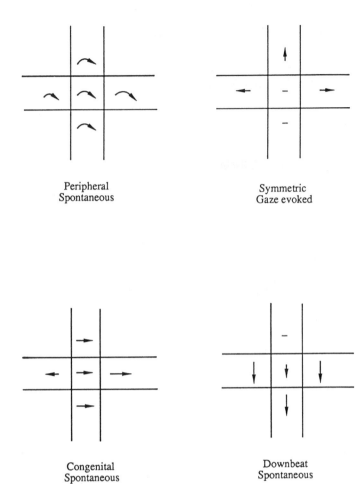

Peripheral
Spontaneous

Symmetric
Gaze evoked

Congenital
Spontaneous

Downbeat
Spontaneous

FIGURE 27 Method for documenting the effect of eye position on nystagmus amplitude and direction. Arrows indicate direction and amplitude of nystagmus (direction of fast component) in each eye position. (From Baloh, RW and Honrubia, V: *Clinical Neurophysiology of the Vestibular System,* ed. 2. F.A. Davis, Philadelphia, 1990, p 119, with permission.)

Table 1 **Differentiating between Different Varieties of Spontaneous Nystagmus**

	Peripheral Vestibular	Central Vestibular	Congenital
Appearance	Combined torsional horizontal	Often pure vertical, horizontal, or torsional	Horizontal, unusual waveform 3–5 Hz
Fixation	Inhibited	Usually little effect	May increase
Gaze	Unidirectional (Alexander's law)	May change direction	May change direction and waveform
Mechanism	Asymmetrical loss of peripheral vestibular tone	Imbalance in central vestibular tone	Imbalance in pursuit or optokinetic tone
Localization	Labyrinth or vestibular	Brain stem or cerebellum	Unknown

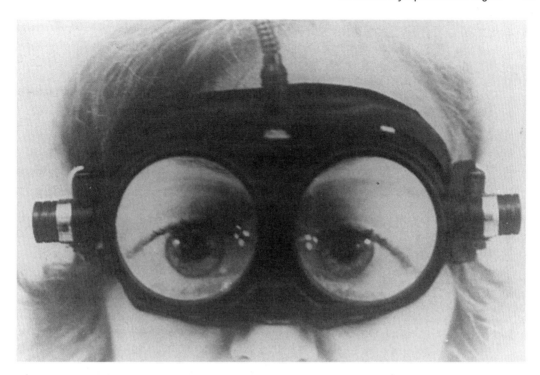

FIGURE 28   Fresnel glasses. (From Baloh, RW and Honrubia, V: *Clinical Neurophysiology of the Vestibular System,* ed. 2. F.A. Davis, Philadelphia, 1990, p. 118, with permission.)

reverse effect (Alexander's law). **Peripheral vestibular nystagmus** is strongly inhibited by fixation. Unless the patient is seen within a few days of the acute episode, spontaneous nystagmus will not be present when fixation is permitted (i.e., on routine examination). In this instance, Fresnel glasses (+30 lenses) are particularly useful for abolishing fixation and uncovering spontaneous vestibular nystagmus (Fig. 28). Acquired persistent spontaneous nystagmus that is not inhibited by fixation (central vestibular nystagmus) indicates a lesion in the brain stem, cerebellum, or both. Central vestibular nystagmus is often purely horizontal or vertical since horizontal and vertical vestibular ocular pathways separate, beginning at the vestibular nuclei.[1] Spontaneous congenital nystagmus is also prominent with fixation, but it can usually be distinguished from acquired central nystagmus based on its long duration, atypical waveforms, and high frequency.

> *Fixation inhibits peripheral vestibular nystagmus but not other spontaneous types.*

Gaze-Evoked Nystagmus

Patients with **gaze-evoked nystagmus** are unable to maintain conjugate eye deviation away from the primary position. The eyes drift back toward the center, and corrective saccades (fast components) are required to maintain the desired gaze position. Gaze-evoked nystagmus is therefore always in the direction of gaze. It

> *Gaze-evoked nystagmus, provoked by eye deviation away from the primary position, is readily observed on routine examination.*

is induced by having the patient fixate on a target 30° to the right, to the left, above, and below the center position. Gaze deviation beyond 30° may result in nystagmus even in normal subjects (so-called **end-point nystagmus**). Gaze-evoked nystagmus is prominent with fixation and is therefore readily observed on routine examination. The site of abnormality can be anywhere from the neuromuscular junction to the multiple brain centers controlling conjugate gaze (Table 2).

Symmetrical gaze-evoked nystagmus (equal amplitude to the right and left) is most commonly produced by ingestion of drugs such as phenobarbital, phenytoin, alcohol, and diazepam. With these agents, high-frequency, small-amplitude nystagmus (usually less than a degree in amplitude) is found in all directions of gaze. The amplitude of the nystagmus is roughly correlated with the drug level in the blood.

Asymmetrical horizontal gaze-evoked nystagmus always indicates a structural brain lesion.

Asymmetrical horizontal gaze-evoked nystagmus always indicates a structural brain lesion. When it is caused by a focal lesion of the brain stem or cerebellum, the larger-amplitude nystagmus is usually directed toward the side of the lesion. Large cerebellopontine angle tumors commonly produce asymmetrical gaze-evoked nystagmus from compression of the brain stem and cerebellum (Bruns' nystagmus).[18]

Rebound nystagmus is a type of gaze-evoked nystagmus that either disappears or reverses direction as the lateral gaze position is held. When the eyes return to the primary position, another burst of nystagmus occurs in the direction of the return saccade. Thus, the patient may have a transient primary position nystagmus in either direction. Rebound nystagmus occurs in patients

Table 2   Differentiating Between Different Varieties of Gaze Nystagmus

	Symmetrical (Gaze Paretic)	Asymmetrical (Bruns' Nystagmus)	Rebound	Dissociated	Congenital
Appearance	Small amplitude, equal in all directions	Larger amplitude, with gaze toward side of lesion	Decays as position is held, transient in primary position	Larger amplitude in abducting eye	Conjugate, high-frequency, variable waveform
Mechanism	Impaired gaze holding	Impaired gaze holding plus tonic bias	Unknown	Impaired gaze holding and delayed transmission through MLF*	Unknown
Localization	Neural integrator (brain stem), myoneural junction, nonspecific	Unilateral or asymmetrical involvement of brain stem, cerebellum, or both	Cerebellum (probably flocculus)	MLF	Unknown

*MLF = medial longitudinal fasciculus.

with cerebellar atrophy and focal structural lesions of the cerebellum; it is the only variety of nystagmus thought to be specific for cerebellar involvement.[19]

The most common variety of **dissociated nystagmus** results from lesions of the medial longitudinal fasciculus (MLF), so-called **internuclear ophthalmoplegia**. With horizontal gaze deviation, the adducting eye lags and develops a low-amplitude "rounded" nystagmus, while the abducting eye develops a large-amplitude nystagmus with a characteristic "sharp-peaked" waveform. Patients with myasthenia gravis may develop a similar type of dissociated nystagmus (so-called **pseudo-MLF nystagmus**), but unlike true MLF nystagmus, their nystagmus progressively increases in amplitude as the gaze position is maintained.

Some varieties of **congenital nystagmus** occur only on lateral gaze, but as with primary position congenital nystagmus, the long history, high frequency, and characteristic waveforms easily distinguish it from other varieties of gaze-evoked nystagmus.[20]

Positional Nystagmus

Two general types of positional nystagmus can be identified on the basis of nystagmus regularity: static and paroxysmal.[1] **Static positional nystagmus** is unrelated to the speed of the position change and can occur in the supine, right lateral, or left lateral position. This type of positional nystagmus persists as long as the position is held. **Paroxysmal positional nystagmus** (also called **positioning nystagmus**), on the other hand, is induced by a rapid position change, either from the erect sitting position to a supine head-hanging left, center, or right position or from the supine to head-right or head-left position. It is initially high in frequency but rapidly dissipates within 30 seconds to 1 minute.

Static positional nystagmus, persisting as long as the particular position is held, most often occurs with peripheral vestibular disorders. If fixation does not suppress the nystagmus, the lesion may be central.

Static positional nystagmus is often not associated with vertigo and is often seen only with the aid of Fresnel lenses to inhibit fixation. It may be unidirectional in all positions or may change direction in different positions. Both direction-changing and direction-fixed static positional nystagmus occur most commonly with peripheral vestibular disorders, but both also can occur with central lesions. As with spontaneous nystagmus, however, lack of suppression with fixation and signs of associated brain stem dysfunction suggest a central lesion.

The most common variety of paroxysmal positional nystagmus (so-called **benign paroxysmal positional nystagmus**) is induced by the Dix-Hallpike positioning test (Fig. 29). After the patient is rapidly moved from the sitting to the head-hanging position, there is a brief latency (3 to 10 seconds), followed by a burst of torsional vertical nystagmus that rarely lasts longer than 30 seconds.[21] The upper pole of the eye beats toward the ground and the main linear component beats upward in the head (i.e., toward the forehead). Benign paroxysmal positional nystagmus is usually prominent in only one head-hanging position, and a lesser burst of nystagmus occurs in the reverse direction when the patient moves back to the sitting position. Another key feature is that the

Paroxysmal positional nystagmus, induced by certain rapid position changes, dissipates in less than 1 minute. If it has no latency and if repeated positioning does not decrease its amplitude and duration, a brain stem or cerebellar lesion may be responsible.

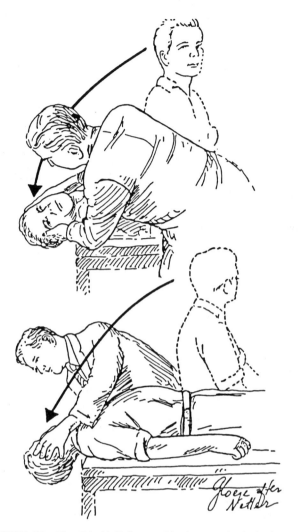

FIGURE 29 The Dix-Hallpike positioning test for inducing paroxysmal positional (positioning) nystagmus. The patient is taken rapidly from the sitting position to the head-hanging position.

patient experiences severe vertigo with initial positioning, but with repeated positioning, vertigo and nystagmus rapidly diminish (fatigue). This type of paroxysmal positional nystagmus is specific for the posterior canal variant of benign positional vertigo (see Chapter 10).

Paroxysmal positional nystagmus can also result from brain stem and cerebellar lesions. This type does not decrease in amplitude or duration with repeated positioning, does not have a clear latency, and usually lasts longer than 30 seconds. The direction is unpredictable and may be different in different positions. It is often purely vertical with the fast phase directed downward (toward the cheeks). Features that distinguish between different types of paroxysmal positional nystagmus are summarized in Table 3.

Table 3   Differentiating between Peripheral and Central Paroxysmal Positional Nystagmus

	Peripheral	Central
Appearance	Torsional upbeat or horizontal geotropic	Pure vertical, usually downbeat
Latency	Usual	Unusual
Fatigability	Usual	Unusual
Mechanism	Debris moving in semicircular canal	Damage to central vestibulo-ocular pathways
Localization	Posterior or horizontal semicircular canal	Brain stem or cerebellum

Hyperventilation-Induced Nystagmus

Hyperventilation can induce a near-faint dizziness in anyone, particularly in anxious patients, but hyperventilation-induced nystagmus is rare.[22] Patients with compressive lesions of the vestibular nerve, such as with an acoustic neuroma or cholesteatoma, or with demyelination of the vestibular nerve root entry zone may develop nystagmus after hyperventilation. Presumably metabolic changes associated with hyperventilation trigger the partially damaged nerve to fire inappropriately. Hyperventilation-induced nystagmus has also rarely been associated with labyrinthitis or perilymph fistula.

Head-Shaking Nystagmus

Patients with a compensated vestibular imbalance due to either peripheral or central lesions may develop a transient spontaneous nystagmus after vigorous head shaking.[23] The test is performed by having the patient shake the head back and forth in the horizontal plane as fast as possible for approximately 10 cycles. Spontaneous nystagmus after head shaking is abnormal, indicating an imbalance within the vestibulo-ocular pathways. With unilateral peripheral vestibular lesions, the abnormal side is in the direction of the slow phase. The results of vertical head shaking are more difficult to interpret because some normal subjects will have transient vertical nystagmus after vertical head shaking.

Nystagmus after vigorous horizontal head shaking indicates an imbalance within the vestibulo-ocular pathways.

Skew Deviation

Skew deviation is a vertical malalignment of the eyes that cannot be explained on the basis of an ocular muscle palsy.[17] It results from an imbalance in tonic signals within the otolith-ocular reflex pathways. Patients with a skew deviation complain of vertical diplopia. There also usually is a cyclorotation (ocular counterroll) of both eyes associated with an illusion of tilt of the visual

Vertical malalignment of the eyes, when accompanied by ocular counterrolling and head tilt, indicates a lesion in the otolith-ocular pathway. Whether the higher or the lower eye is on the side of the lesion depends on how far along the pathway the lesion is.

world.[24] The head may also be tilted, toward the side of the lower eye. Skew deviation, ocular counterrolling, and head tilt together form the **ocular-tilt response** (Fig. 30).

Skew deviation is best detected at the bedside with the **alternate cover-uncover** test.[17] The examiner switches the cover from one eye to the other while looking for vertical corrective eye movements. Skew deviations tend to be relatively commitant; that is, the degree of misalignment changes little with different directions of gaze. The ocular-tilt reaction can occur with lesions anywhere in the otolith-ocular pathway, including the labyrinth, vestibular nerve, vestibular nucleus, medial longitudinal fasciculus, and midbrain.[24] As shown in Figure 30, with peripheral and vestibular nuclear lesions (such as immediately after a vestibular nerve section or with Wallenberg syndrome) the lower eye is on the side of the lesion. The otolith-ocular pathway crosses at the level of the vestibular nucleus, and with lesions above the decussation (such as a lesion of the midbrain), the higher eye is on the side of the lesion.

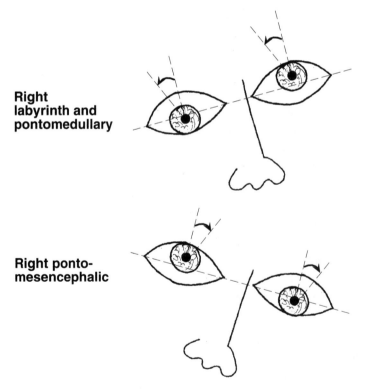

Right labyrinth and pontomedullary

Right ponto-mesencephalic

FIGURE 30   Ocular-tilt responses associated with lesions at different locations within the peripheral and central vestibular pathways. The ocular-tilt reaction consists of a head tilt toward the side of the lower eye, a skew deviation with one eye higher than the other, and counter roll (torsion) of both eyes, with the top poles rolling toward the side of the lower eye. With lesions of the labyrinth and pontomedullary regions, the ipsilateral eye is down; it is up with lesions in the pontomesencephalic region.

References

1. Baloh RW, and Honrubia V: Clinical Neurophysiology of the Vestibular System, ed 2. F.A. Davis, Philadelphia, 1990.
2. Yates BJ, Grelot L, Kerman L, et al: The organization of vestibular inputs to nucleus solitarius and adjacent structures in the cat. Am J Physiol 267:R974, 1994.
3. Yates BJ, Siniaia MS, and Miller AD: Descending pathways necessary for vestibular influences on sympathetic and inspiratory outflow. Am J Physiol 286:R1381, 1995.
4. Fife TD, and Baloh RW: Disequilibrium of unknown cause in older people. Ann Neurol 34:694, 1993.
5. Drachmann, DA, and Hart CW: An approach to the dizzy patient. Neurology 22:323, 1972.
6. Hess K, Gresty M, and Leech J: Clinical and theoretical aspects of head movement dependent oscillopsia (HMDO). J Neurol 219:151, 1978.
7. Hess K: Vestibulotoxic drugs and other causes of acquired bilateral peripheral vestibulopathy. In Baloh RW, and Halmagyi GM (eds): Disorders of the Vestibular System. Oxford University Press, New York, 1996.
8. Money KE: Motion sickness. Physiol Rev 50:1, 1970.
9. Takeda N, and Matsunaga T: Neurochemical basis of motion sickness and its treatment and prevention. In Baloh RW, and Halmagyi GM (eds): Disorders of the Vestibular System. Oxford University Press, New York, 1996.
10. Dichgans J, and Brandt T: Visual-vestibular integration and motion perception. In Bizzi E, and Dichgans F (eds): Cerebral Control of Eye Movements and Motion Perception. S. Karger, Basel, 1972.
11. Johnson WH, and Jongkees LBW: Motion sickness. In Kornhuber HH (ed): Handbook of Sensory Physiology, vol. VI, part 2. Springer-Verlag, New York, 1974.
12. Brown JJ, and Baloh RW: Persistent mal de debarquement syndrome: A motion induced subjective disorder. Am J Otolaryngol 8:219, 1987.
13. Peitersen E: Measurement of vestibulo-spinal responses in man. In Kornhuber HH (ed): Handbook of Sensory Physiology, vol. VI, part 2. Springer-Verlag, New York, 1974.
14. Halmagyi GM, and Curthoys IS: A clinical sign of canal paresis. Arch Neurol 45:737, 1988.
15. Longridge NS, and Mallinson AI: The dynamic illegible E (DIE) test: A simple technique for assessing the vestibulo-ocular reflex to overcome vestibular pathology. Can J Otolaryngol 16:97, 1987.
16. Burgio DL, Blakeley BW, and Myers SF: The high-frequency oscillopsia test. J Vestib Res 2:221, 1992.
17. Leigh RJ, and Zee DS: The Neurology of Eye Movements, ed 2. F.A. Davis, Philadelphia, 1991.
18. Baloh RW, Konrad HR, Dirks D, and Honrubia V: Cerebellar-pontine angle tumors: Results of quantitative vestibulo-ocular testing. Arch Neurol 33:507, 1976.
19. Hood JD, Kayan A, and Leech J: Rebound nystagmus. Brain 96:507, 1973.
20. Spooner JS, and Baloh RW: Eye movement fatigue in myasthenia gravis. Neurology 29:29, 1979.
21. Baloh RW, Sakala SM, and Honrubia V: Benign paroxysmal positional nystagmus. Am J Otolaryngol 1:1, 1979.
22. Zee DS, and Fletcher WA: Bedside examination. In Baloh RW, and Halmagyi GM (eds): Disorders of the Vestibular System. Oxford University Press, New York, 1996.
23. Hain TC, and Spinder J: Head-shaking nystagmus. In Sharpe JA, and Barber HO (eds): The Vestibulo-Ocular Reflex and Vertigo. Raven Press, New York, 1993.
24. Brandt T, and Dieterich M: Vestibular syndromes in the roll plane: Topographic diagnosis from brain stem to cortex. Ann Neurol 36:337, 1994.

6

Evaluation of Vestibular Function

Chapter Outline

Current tests of vestibular function concentrate on the horizontal semicircular canal – ocular reflex because it is the easiest reflex to stimulate (calorically and rotationally) and to record (using electro-oculography). Tests of the other vestibulo-ocular reflexes (vertical semicircular canal and otolith) and of the vestibulospinal reflexes have yet to be shown as useful in the clinical setting.[1]

COLD CALORIC TEST

The caloric test uses a nonphysiological stimulus to induce endolymphatic flow in the horizontal semicircular canal and, thus, horizontal nystagmus, by creating a temperature gradient from one side of the canal to the other.[2] With a cold caloric stimulus, the column of endolymph nearest the middle ear falls because of its increased density. This causes the cupula to deviate away from the utricle (utriculofugal flow) and produces horizontal nystagmus with the fast phase directed away from the stimulated ear

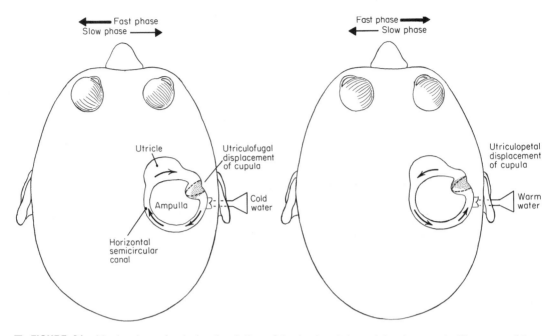

FIGURE 31 Mechanism of caloric stimulation of the horizontal semicircular canals. The eyes of the comatose patient deviate in the direction of the slow phase (as shown).

(Fig. 31). A warm stimulus produces the opposite effect, causing utriculopetal endolymph flow and nystagmus directed toward the stimulated ear (COWS—cold opposite, warm same). Because of its ready availability, ice water (approximately 0°C) is usually used for bedside caloric testing.[3] To bring the horizontal canal into the vertical plane, the patient lies in the supine position with the head tilted 30° forward. One begins by placing 0.5 mL of ice water up against the tympanic membrane on each side using a 1-mL syringe. If no response is elicited, larger volumes of ice water can be used (up to 10 mL). In a comatose patient, only a slow tonic deviation toward the side of stimulation is observed. In normal subjects, the duration and speed of induced nystagmus varies greatly, depending on the size of the external canal, the thickness of the temporal bone, the circulation to the temporal bone, and the subject's ability to use fixation to suppress the nystagmus. Asymmetry of more than 20% in nystagmus duration suggests a lesion on the side of the decreased response. This should always be confirmed, however, with standard bithermal caloric testing and electronystagmography (discussed later).

Asymmetrical duration of nystagmus on cold caloric testing suggests a lesion on the side of the decreased response.

BEDSIDE ROTATIONAL TESTING

Qualitative rotational testing of the horizontal vestibulo-ocular reflex can be performed at the bedside by using a swivel chair. The patient is given approximately 10 revolutions in 20 seconds and then suddenly stopped, facing the observer. The duration of postrotatory nystagmus in each direction is then measured. Postrotatory nystagmus generally lasts about 20 seconds in normal subjects, but intersubject variability is large. Much of this variability can be traced to the difficulty in manually maintaining constant velocity and then a uniform sudden deceleration. As with the ice water caloric test, this type of qualitative testing provides only gross information about the presence and symmetry of vestibulo-ocular function.

The fixation-suppression test can be performed with the patient sitting in the same swivel chair, but in this case the patient extends one arm rigidly and attempts to fixate on the extended thumb while the entire body is rotated back and forth en bloc (about 1 cycle in 2 seconds). Normal subjects can completely suppress their vestibulo-ocular reflex, keeping their eyes fixed in the center of the orbit. Nystagmus indicates a central lesion, often involving the cerebellum.

ELECTRONYSTAGMOGRAPHY

Electronystagmography (ENG) is a technique for recording eye movements based on the corneal retinal potential (Fig. 32).[1] The pigmented layer of the retina maintains a negative potential with regard to the surrounding tissue by means of active ion transport. Because of the sclera's insulating properties, the cornea is positive in relation to the retina. Thus, each eye is like a small battery with a surrounding electromagnetic field. In relation to a remote electrode, an electrode placed near the eye becomes more positive when the eye rotates toward it and less positive when the eye rotates away from it. Recordings are usually made with a three-electrode system using differential amplifiers. Two active electrodes are placed on each side of the eye and the reference (ground) electrode is placed somewhere remote from the eyes, usually on the forehead. The two active electrodes measure a potential change of equal amplitude but opposite direction. The difference in potential between these electrodes is amplified and used to control a pen-writing recorder or similar device to produce a permanent record. Since the differential amplifiers monitor the difference in voltage between the two active electrodes, remote electric signals (such as electromyographic or electroencephalographic signals) that arrive at the electrodes with approximately equal amplitude and phase are canceled out.

By convention, for horizontal recordings, eye movements to the right are displayed so that they produce upward pen deflection, and those to the left produce downward deflection (Fig. 33). For vertical recordings, upward eye movements produce upward deflections, and vice versa. Vertical recordings are particularly prone to eyelid movement artifacts, however. Calibration is necessary to interpret ENG recordings, so that a standard angle of eye deviation is represented by a known amplitude of pen deflection. Calibration is performed by having the patient maintain his or her gaze on a series of dots or lights 10 to 20° on each side of,

Normal subjects typically have nystagmus if they are rapidly rotated on a swivel chair and then suddenly stopped.

ENG uses the eye's corneal retinal potential to produce a record of eye movements.

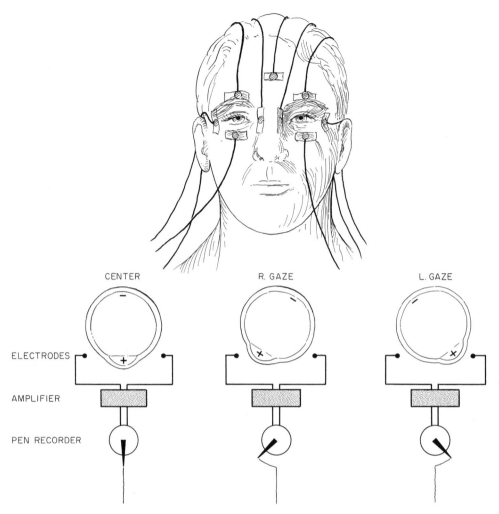

CENTER   R. GAZE   L. GAZE

ELECTRODES

AMPLIFIER

PEN RECORDER

■ **FIGURE 32**   Principle of electronystagmography (ENG).

With ENG, you can quantify the magnitude of nystagmus and assess the effect of loss of fixation by recording eye movements in a dark room.

and above and below, the central fixation point. Once this relationship is established, the amplitude, duration, and velocity of recorded eye movements can be easily calculated.

With ENG, one can quantify the slow component velocity, frequency, and amplitude of pathological or physiological nystagmus and the changes in these measurements brought about by loss of fixation (either with eyes closed or eyes open in darkness). Changes from loss of fixation are particularly important, since peripheral vestibular nystagmus often is present only when fixation is inhibited (as in Fig. 33, right side). As a rule, nystagmus with fixation (nystagmus seen on routine neurologic examination) disappears within a few days after the occurrence of an acute peripheral vestibular lesion. By contrast, peripheral vestibular nystagmus may be recorded with eyes closed or with eyes open in darkness (i.e., without fixation) for as long as 5 to 10 years after such a lesion. In some patients, vestibular nystagmus emerges only when they are distracted (e.g., when performing serial 7 subtractions from 100).

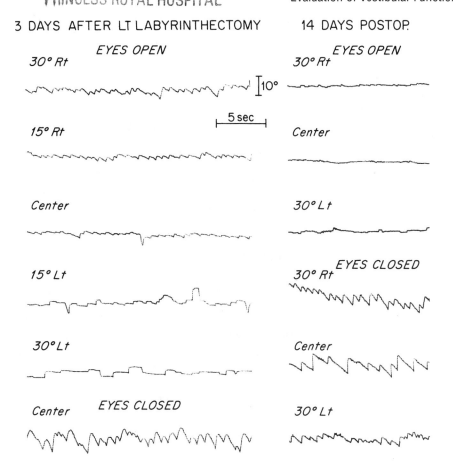

FIGURE 33 ENG recordings of right beating spontaneous nystagmus 3 days and 14 days after the patient underwent a left labyrinthectomy. Nystagmus with eyes open disappeared by 14 days, but nystagmus with eyes closed remains prominent. (Adapted from Baloh, RW: Pathologic nystagmus: A classification based on electro-oculographic recordings. Bull Los Angeles Neurol Soc 41:120, 1976, with permission.)

A standard ENG test battery should include tests in three major areas: (1) pathological nystagmus, (2) vestibulo-ocular reflex function, and (3) visual ocular control. Examination for pathological nystagmus requires a systematic study of:

- Changes in fixation (eyes opened fixating, eyes opened in darkness, eyes closed)
- Changes in gaze position (30° left, right, up, and down)
- Changes in head position (supine, head-hanging, and lateral positions)

Recordings can also be made after changing pressure in the external ear canal (fistula test), after hyperventilation, and after head shaking.

Vestibulo-ocular reflex function is tested with bithermal caloric stimulation and physiological rotational stimuli. Examination of visual ocular control includes tests of saccades, smooth pursuit, and optokinetic nystagmus (discussed later).

> *An ENG test battery typically includes tests for pathological nystagmus, vestibulo-ocular reflexes, and visual ocular control.*

BITHERMAL CALORIC TESTING

Bithermal caloric testing has several major advantages:

- Both utriculopetal and utriculofugal endolymph flow are serially induced in each horizontal semicircular canal.
- The caloric stimulus is reproducible from patient to patient.
- The magnitude of response is accurately measured.
- The test is tolerated by most patients.

The major limitation is the need for ENG equipment and constant temperature baths and plumbing to maintain continuous circulation of the water through the infusion hose.

Technique

To perform bithermal caloric testing, each ear is irrigated for a fixed duration (30 to 40 seconds) at a constant flow rate of water that is 7° below body temperature (30°C) and 7° above body temperature (44°C). The patient lies in the supine position with head tilted 30° forward and eyes open in total darkness. ENG is used to measure the **slow component velocity (SCV)** of the induced nystagmus (Fig. 34). Computers can rapidly calculate the SCV of each beat of nystagmus and generate curves of SCV versus time, such as those shown in Figure 35. Maximum SCV is the most sensitive measure of the caloric response.[1]

The four responses of a bithermal caloric test are routinely compared using two standard formulas (Fig. 35). The **vestibular paresis** formula

$$\frac{(R30° + R44°) - (L30° + L44°)}{R30° + R44° + L30° + L44°} \times 100$$

compares the right-sided responses with the left-sided responses, and the **directional preponderance** formula

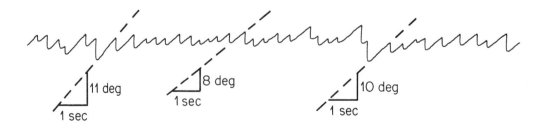

FIGURE 34 ENG recording of caloric-induced nystagmus. The slope of the slow phase gives the slow component velocity (SCV).

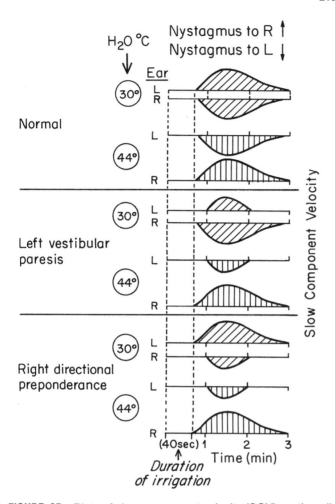

FIGURE 35 Plots of slow component velocity (SCV) vs. time, illustrating three characteristic responses to bithermal caloric testing. Normal: Peak SCV and duration are symmetrical. Left vestibular paresis: Peak SCV and duration are decreased when the left ear is stimulated. Right directional preponderance: Peak SCV and duration of nystagmus to the right (L30 and R44) are greater than peak SCV and duration of nystagmus to the left (R30 and L44).

$$\frac{(R30° + L44°) - (R44° + L30°)}{R30° + L44° + R44° + L30°} \times 100$$

compares nystagmus to the right with nystagmus to the left in the same subject. In both of these formulas, the difference in response is reported as a percentage of the total response. This is important because the absolute magnitude of caloric response depends on several factors, including age.[4] Dividing by the total response normalizes the measurements to remove the large variability in absolute magnitude of normal caloric responses. In our laboratory, the upper normal value for vestibular paresis is 25%

Differences found on bithermal caloric testing are reported as percentages of the total response to eliminate the variability in the absolute magnitude of normal responses.

and that for directional preponderance is 30% (using maximum SCV in the above equations).[1]

Interpreting Test Results

A vestibular paresis on bithermal caloric testing indicates a peripheral vestibular lesion, but a directional preponderance is nonlocalizing.

Generally, a significant vestibular paresis on bithermal caloric testing indicates a peripheral vestibular lesion (including the nerve root entry zone), whereas a significant directional preponderance is nonlocalizing (i.e., it can occur with both peripheral and central lesions). Directional preponderance is often associated with spontaneous nystagmus, in which the velocity of the slow component of the spontaneous nystagmus adds to that of the caloric-induced nystagmus in the same direction and subtracts from that of the caloric-induced nystagmus in the opposite direction.

The vestibular paresis and directional preponderance formulas are of little use in evaluating patients with bilateral vestibular lesions whose caloric responses are symmetrically depressed. Because of the wide range of normal values for maximum SCV (5 to 60°/sec in our laboratory), the patient's value may decrease several-fold before falling below the normal range.[2] Serial measurements in the same patient are needed if one hopes to identify early bilateral vestibular impairment such as that produced by ototoxic drugs.

Serial measurements are needed to identify early bilateral vestibular impairment.

Because of the wide range, it is unusual to find caloric responses that exceed the upper normal range. Lesions of the cerebellum occasionally can lead to bilateral increased caloric responses, apparently owing to the loss of the normal inhibitory influence of the cerebellum on the vestibular nuclei.

ROTATIONAL TESTING

Rotational tests of the vestibulo-ocular reflexes are not widely used as part of the routine vestibular examination because rotational stimuli affect both labyrinths simultaneously, unlike the selective stimulation possible with caloric tests. They also require expensive, bulky equipment to generate precise rotational stimuli.[1]

Rotational tests do have several advantages, however. Multiple graded stimuli can be applied in a relatively short period of time, and rotational testing is usually less bothersome to patients than is caloric testing. Unlike caloric testing, a rotational stimulus to the semicircular canals is unrelated to physical features of the external ear or temporal bone, so that a more exact relationship between stimulus and response is possible.

Technique

The patient is seated in a chair that rotates about its vertical axis. The head is fixed so that angular rotation occurs in the plane of one of the semicircular canal pairs (usually with the head tilted 30° forward, so that rotation occurs in the plane of the horizontal canals). The patient's eyes are opened in complete darkness, and the induced nystagmus is recorded with ENG. The **gain** of the response, defined as the peak slow component eye velocity divided by the peak chair velocity, is calculated for nystagmus in each direction. Sinusoidal and step (impulse) changes in angular velocity are routinely used (Fig. 36). For sinusoidal stimuli, normal gain

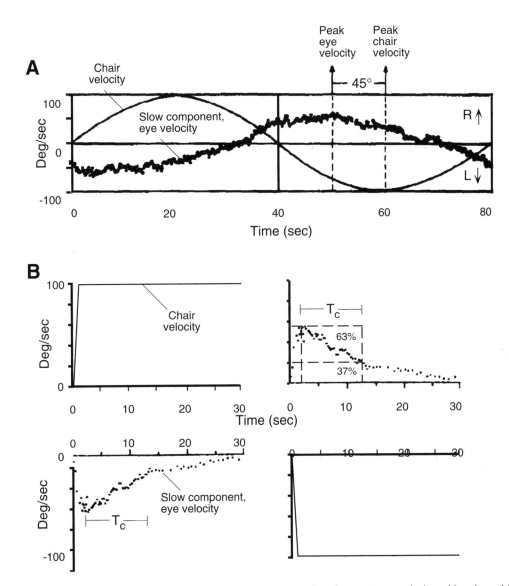

FIGURE 36 Plots of slow component eye velocity versus time for nystagmus induced by sinusoidal angular rotation in the horizontal plane at 0.0125 Hz and a peak velocity of 100°/sec (*A*) and by step changes in angular velocity of 100°/sec occurring with an acceleration of approximately 140°/sec^2 (*B*). Subject is seated on a motorized rotating chair with eyes open in darkness. Eye movements are recorded with ENG. Fast components are identified and removed and slow component eye velocity is measured every 20 msec. The gain of the response (peak slow component eye velocity ÷ peak chair velocity) is about 0.6 for both types of stimulation. The phase lead with sinusoidal stimulation (*A*) is the difference in timing between the peak eye velocity and peak chair velocity (in this case 45°). The time constant (T$_c$) is the time required for the response to decay to 37% of its initial value (about 10 seconds in *B*).

Table 4   **Normal Values for Rotational Testing with Sinusoidal and Step Stimuli**

Sine Frequency (Hz)	Gain	Phase (°)
0.0125	0.40 ± 0.07	39 ± 7
0.05	0.50 ± 0.15	10 ± 4
0.40	0.59 ± 0.09	0
1.0	0.81 ± 0.19	0
1.5	1.01 ± 0.12	0
Step (°/Sec)	**Gain**	**Time Constant (Seconds)**
100	0.63 ± 0.18	12.2 ± 3.6

varies with frequency, being approximately 0.5 at low frequencies (e.g., 0.05 Hz) and near 1.0 for higher frequencies (>1 Hz) (Table 4). For step changes in angular velocity, the normal gain is about 0.65 (see Table 4).

For sinusoidal rotational testing, the **phase** of the response refers to the timing between the maximum velocity of the head and the maximum velocity of the slow components of nystagmus. This is usually calculated by performing a frequency analysis (Fourier analysis) of the SCV trace and comparing the phase of the fundamental frequency to the phase of the head velocity trace.[5] In normal subjects, there is a phase lead of eye velocity relative to head velocity at low frequencies (approximately 45° at 0.01 Hz, as illustrated in Fig. 36) but not at higher frequencies (>0.2 Hz) (see Table 4). For step rotational testing, the **time constant** refers to the time it takes for nystagmus SCV to decay to 63% of the peak value (see Fig. 36 and Table 4).

Interpreting Rotational Test Results

Rotational testing can identify complete unilateral loss of vestibular function, but it's less useful for identifying partial unilateral lesions.

Rotational testing is good for evaluating patients with bilateral peripheral vestibular lesions.

Patients with complete unilateral loss of vestibular function have asymmetrical gain (decreased with head rotation toward the abnormal side) best identified with high-velocity step stimuli. Patients who show a partial unilateral vestibular paresis on caloric stimulation may have symmetrical rotation-induced nystagmus, however, since the remaining intact labyrinth is able to compensate for the damaged side.[6] For this reason, rotational testing is not particularly useful for identifying early partial unilateral peripheral vestibular lesions. With compensation, the asymmetry of rotational-induced nystagmus disappears within a few weeks, but the increased phase lead and shortened time constant remain indefinitely.[7] An increase in the low-frequency phase lead and shortening of the time constant are nonspecific findings that can occur with both peripheral (unilateral and bilateral) and central vestibular lesions.

Rotational testing is very useful for evaluating patients with bilateral peripheral vestibular lesions (e.g., ototoxic exposure), since both labyrinths are stimulated simultaneously and the degree of remaining function is accurately quantified.[8] Because the variance associated with normal rotational responses is less than that associated with caloric responses, diminished function is identified earlier.

Patients with absent caloric responses may show decreased, but measurable, rotation-induced nystagmus, particularly at higher stimulus velocities. The ability to identify remaining vestibular function, even if minimal, is an important advantage of rotational testing, particularly when the physician is contemplating ablative surgery or monitoring the effects of ototoxic drugs.

Artifactually diminished caloric responses occasionally occur in patients with angular, narrow external canals or with highly pneumatized temporal bones. Because a rotational stimulus is unrelated to these factors, rotation-induced nystagmus is normal in such patients.

Like normal subjects, patients with peripheral vestibular lesions can suppress physiological vestibular nystagmus when they are rotated with a fixation point. Rotational stimuli are ideally suited for evaluating fixation suppression of the vestibulo-ocular reflex, since the same precise stimulus can be presented on repeated occasions with and without fixation. Impaired fixation suppression of rotation-induced nystagmus is nearly always associated with abnormal smooth pursuit.[9]

Rotational testing is better than caloric testing at identifying minimal vestibular function.

Autorotational testing can be used to monitor vestibular function at the bedside in patients receiving potentially ototoxic drugs.

AUTOROTATIONAL TESTING

For head-only rotational testing, the patient moves the head voluntarily while head movement is monitored with a rotational velocity sensor affixed to a lightweight helmet, and eye movements are recorded with ENG.[10] The main advantage of head-only rotational testing is that bulky, expensive rotational equipment is not required, so that the testing potentially can be performed at the bedside. The disadvantages include a limited range of stimulus magnitude and frequency; difficulty in separating small saccades from compensatory slow movements, owing to the poor signal-to-noise ratio of ENG; and the ability of self-generated volitional movements to partially compensate for peripheral vestibular loss.

Subjects can typically rotate their head back and forth between about 0.5 and 3 Hz. Data analysis proceeds in the same manner as for conventional rotational testing, with measures of gain, phase, and symmetry for different frequencies of head rotation. With ENG, head-only rotational testing can reliably assess only the horizontal vestibulo-ocular reflex (VOR); blink artifacts confound assessment of the vertical VOR. Head-only rotational testing is primarily useful for identifying and following the progress of bilateral vestibular loss associated with ototoxicity drugs.

TESTS OF VISUAL-OCULAR CONTROL

Along with the vestibulo-ocular reflexes, two visually controlled ocular stabilizing systems produce versional eye movements—the saccadic and the smooth pursuit systems.[11] The **saccade system** responds to a retinal position error to bring a peripheral target to the fovea in the shortest possible time. The **smooth pursuit system** maintains gaze on a moving target by generating a continuous match of eye and target velocity. **Optokinetic nystagmus** is a form of smooth pursuit in which the eye-tracking motion in one direction is periodically interrupted by corrective saccades in the opposite direction to relocate the gaze on new targets coming into the visual field.

Technique

Saccadic eye movements are induced by having the patient follow a target moving in a stepwise pattern. Pursuit eye movements are similarly induced using a sinusoidal pattern. For optokinetic testing, a striped pattern is moved across the patient's visual field in a clockwise and counterclockwise direction.

With ENG, features of these visually controlled eye movements can be accurately measured and the results compared with normative data (Fig. 37). One typically measures the peak veloc-

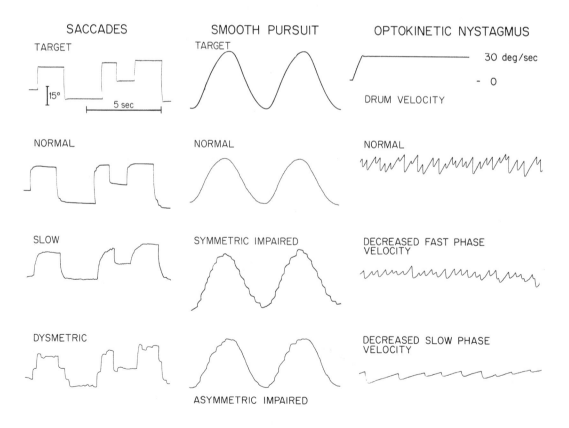

FIGURE 37 ENG recordings of normal and abnormal saccades, smooth pursuit, and optokinetic nystagmus. See text for interpretation of abnormalities.

ity, accuracy, and reaction time of saccadic eye movements. For pursuit and optokinetic nystagmus, the tracking eye velocity is compared with the target or optokinetic drum velocity.

Interpreting Visual Tracking Test Results

Abnormalities of visual ocular control can be very useful for localizing lesions within the central nervous system (Table 5).[3] With one exception, peripheral vestibular lesions do not impair visual ocular control. The exception is that, after an acute unilateral labyrinthine or vestibular nerve lesion, smooth pursuit and optokinetic slow component velocity will be transiently decreased to the contralateral side (i.e., in the direction of the spontaneous nystagmus). The asymmetry in smooth pursuit and optokinetic nystagmus disappears in a few weeks, despite the persistence of vestibular nystagmus in darkness.

Slowing of saccadic eye movements results from lesions anywhere from the horizontal gaze centers in the paramedian pontine reticular formation and the vertical gaze centers in the pretectum to the extraocular motoneurons, nerves, and muscles. Lesions involving these structures and interconnecting pathways slow both voluntary saccades and fast components of nystagmus (involuntary saccades) (as illustrated in Fig. 37). Reversible saccade slowing is produced in normal subjects by fatigue and by ingestion of alcohol or tranquilizers. Saccade slowing produced by myasthenia gravis increases with fatigue and is reversed with edrophonium.[12] Lesions of the medial longitudinal fasciculus (MLF) result in slowing of adducting saccades made by the medial rectus

Abnormal saccades, smooth pursuit, or optokinetic nystagmus can be used to localize lesions in the central nervous system.

Alcohol, tranquilizers, or fatigue can impair saccades and smooth pursuit.

Table 5   **Summary of Visual Ocular Control Abnormalities Produced by Focal Neurological Lesions**

Location of Lesion	Saccades	Smooth Pursuit	Optokinetic Nystagmus
Unilateral peripheral vestibular	Normal	Transient contralateral impairment	Transient contralateral decreased SCV*
Cerebellopontine angle	Ipsilateral dysmetria†	Progressive ipsilateral or bilateral impairment	Progressive ipsilateral or bilateral decreased SCV
Diffuse cerebellar	Bilateral dysmetria	Bilateral impairment	Bilateral decreased SCV
Intrinsic brain stem	Decreased maximum velocity, increased delay time	Ipsilateral or bilateral impairment	Ipsilateral or bilateral decreased SCV, disconjugate
Basal ganglia	Hypometria,‡ increased delay time (bilateral)	Bilateral impairment	Bilateral decreased SCV
Frontoparietal cortex	Contralateral hypometria	Normal	Normal
Parieto-occipital cortex	Normal	Ipsilateral impairment	Ipsilateral decreased SCV

*SCV = Slow component velocity.
†Undershoots and overshoots.
‡Undershoots only.

on the side of the lesion.[13] Occasionally, saccade slowing can be identified with ENG recordings when it is not apparent on clinical examination.

Lesions of the supranuclear saccade control centers are often not associated with saccade slowing but rather with an alteration in the accuracy or initiation (reaction time) of saccades. For example, patients with Parkinson's disease exhibit delayed saccade reaction time and hypometric (too small) voluntary saccades.[14] Impaired accuracy is most prominent with cerebellar lesions. Both overshooting and undershooting of the target occur, requiring several corrective saccades to attain the target position (saccade dysmetria). Lesions of the frontal cortex also affect the accuracy of saccades, with saccades to the contralateral side being hypometric. Vertical saccades are unaffected by unilateral cortical lesions.

Patients with impaired smooth pursuit use frequent corrective saccades to keep up with the target and produce so-called cogwheel or saccadic pursuit (as shown in Fig. 37). The pursuit gain (peak pursuit velocity ÷ peak target velocity) is markedly decreased in such patients. Normal subjects may also intermix saccades with smooth pursuit if the target velocity exceeds the limit of their smooth pursuit system (usually about 60°/sec). With ENG, one can use precise stimulus velocities and accurately measure the pursuit velocity between corrective saccades.

Abnormal smooth pursuit occurs with lesions throughout the nervous system.[3] As with saccadic eye movements, tranquilizers, alcohol, and fatigue impair smooth pursuit in normal subjects. Patients with diffuse cortical disease, basal ganglia disease, and cerebellar disease consistently have bilaterally impaired smooth pursuit. Unilateral lesions of the parietal lobe, cerebellum, brain stem, and cerebellopontine angle usually produce ipsilateral impairment of smooth pursuit.

Since optokinetic nystagmus combines pursuit and saccadic eye movements, lesions that affect either or both of these systems produce abnormal optokinetic nystagmus. Symmetrically decreased slow component velocity occurs with disease of the cortex, diencephalon, brain stem, and cerebellum. As with smooth pursuit, unilateral lesions of the parietal cortex, brain stem, and cerebellum impair optokinetic nystagmus when the stripes move toward the side of the lesion.[15] Patients who cannot generate saccades produce a tonic deviation of the eyes in the direction of the optokinetic stimulus, with absent or small abortive fast components.[16]

POSTUROGRAPHY

Posturography is a way of quantifying postural sway.[17] The simplest method employs a so-called force plate that records the position of a subject's center of pressure during upright stance. The position of the center of pressure, which is a good estimate of the position of the center of mass if the body is moving slowly. The limitations of such devices relate to two areas:

1. The nervous system uses a combination of sensory modalities during the maintenance of upright stance.
2. Static force plates do not yield controlled stimulus-response measures of vestibulospinal function and thus must rely on spontaneous movements of the body.

On average, sway increases as normal subjects grow older and in patients with imbalance regardless of the cause, but measurements of sway on a static force plate have not been very sensitive for identifying balance problems.[18,19]

With a moving force platform, one can move the platform upon which the subject stands and simultaneously move the visual surround. Such **dynamic posturography** devices overcome the limitations of static force platforms by controlling the relative contributions of the visual, somatosensory, and vestibular inputs that are normally used to maintain upright posture. They also incorporate stimulus-response measurements.[17] By coupling the platform to the sway of the subject (**sway referencing**) it is possible to maintain the angle between the foot and the lower leg at a constant value, thereby reducing a major source of somatosensory input to the postural control system.[20] If the subject simultaneously closes his or her eyes or if the movement of the visual enclosure is coupled to body sway, the subject is also deprived of visual information about postural sway. In this way, the influence of the labyrinth on upright posture via the vestibulospinal system can be studied in more or less isolated fashion.

Not surprisingly, patients with bilateral peripheral vestibular loss perform poorly on dynamic posturography when visual and somatosensory signals have been effectively removed. The results are often nonspecific, however, and for some patients may suggest vestibular disease even when it is not present. Patients with unilateral vestibular loss usually perform normally on dynamic posturography.[21] Some neurologic abnormalities, such as cerebellar and basal ganglia disease, also are undetected by dynamic posturography.[22] Nor does dynamic posturography provide localizing information with regard to peripheral or central abnormalities. Although evaluation of this kind of testing is still an active area of research, it seems now that its main use will be as a quantitative measure for following patients' progress, particularly as a research tool to evaluate the effects of specific treatments.

Posturography is not especially useful for localizing lesions, but it may be a helpful measure for following a patient's progress.

References

1. Baloh RW, and Furman JM: Modern vestibular function testing. West J Med 150:59, 1989.
2. Baloh RW, and Honrubia V: Clinical Neurophysiology of the Vestibular System, ed 2. F.A. Davis, Philadelphia, 1990.
3. Eviator A, and Eviator L: A critical look at "cold calorics." Arch Otolaryngol 99:361, 1974.
4. Baloh RW, Solingen L, Sills A, and Honrubia V: Caloric testing. I. Effect of different conditions of ocular fixation. Ann Otol Rhinol Laryngol 86 (Suppl 43):1, 1977.
5. Baloh RW, Langhofer L, Honrubia V, and Yee RD: On-line analysis of eye movements using a digital computer. Aviat Space Environ Med 51:563, 1980.

6. Baloh RW, Sills AW, and Honrubia V: Impulsive and sinusoidal rotatory testing: Clinical and oculographic features. Neurology 41:429, 1979.

7. Jenkins HA: Long-term adaptive changes of the vestibulo-ocular reflex in patients following acoustic neuroma surgery. Laryngoscope 95:1224, 1985.

8. Hess K: Vestibulotoxic drugs and other causes of acquired bilateral peripheral vestibulopathy. In Baloh RW, and Halmagyi GM (eds): Disorders of the Vestibular System. Oxford University Press, New York, 1996.

9. Baloh RW, Yee RD, Jenkins HA, and Honrubia V: Quantitative assessment of visual-vestibular interaction using sinusoidal rotatory stimuli. In Honrubia V, and Brazier AB (eds): Nystagmus and Vertigo. Academic Press, New York, 1982.

10. Fineberg R, O'Leary DP, and Davis LL: Use of active head movements for computerized vestibular testing. Arch Otolaryngol Head Neck Surg 113:1063, 1987.

11. Leigh RJ, and Zee DS: The Neurology of Eye Movements, ed 2. F.A. Davis, Philadelphia, 1991.

12. Baloh RW, and Keesey JC: Saccade fatigue and response to edrophonium for the diagnosis of myasthenia gravis. Ann N Y Acad Sci 274:631, 1976.

13. Baloh RW, Yee RD, and Honrubia V: Internuclear ophthalmoplegia. I. Saccades and dissociated nystagmus. Arch Neurol 35:484, 1978.

14. Bronstein AM, and Rudge P: Vestibular disorders due to multiple sclerosis, Arnold-Chiari malformations, and basal ganglia disorders. In Baloh RW, and Halmagyi GM (eds): Disorders of the Vestibular System. Oxford University Press, New York, 1996.

15. Baloh RW, Yee RD, and Honrubia V: Clinical abnormalities in optokinetic nystagmus. In Lennerstrand G, and Zee D (eds): Functional Basis of Ocular Motility Disorders. Pergamon Press, New York, 1982.

16. Baloh RW, Furman J, and Yee RD: Eye movements in patient with absent voluntary horizontal gaze. Ann Neurol 17:283, 1985.

17. Furman JM: Posturography — Use and limitations. In Baloh RW (ed): Bailliere's Clinical Neurology. International Practice and Research: Neurotology. Bailliere Tindall, London, 1994.

18. Baloh RW, Fife TD, Zwerling L, et al: Comparison of static and dynamic posturography in young and older normal people. J Am Geriatr Soc 42:405, 1994.

19. Baloh RW, Spain S, Socotch TM, et al: Posturography and balance problems in older people. J Am Geriatr Soc 43:1, 1995.

20. Nashner LM, Horak FB, and Diener HC: Scaling postural response amplitudes: Normals and patients with cerebellar deficits. Neurology 37 (Suppl 1):281, 1987.

21. Fetter M, Diener HC, and Dichgans J: Recovery of postural control after an acute unilateral vestibular lesion in humans. J Vestib Res 1:373, 1991.

22. Fetter M, and Dichgans J: Vestibular tests in evolution. II. Posturography. In Baloh RW, and Halmagyi GM (eds): Disorders of the Vestibular System. Oxford University Press, New York, 1996.

7

Evaluation of Hearing

Chapter Outline

TYPES OF HEARING LOSS

Hearing loss can be classified as conductive, sensorineural, or central based on the anatomical site of pathology. Important details in the history that can help differentiate between different types of hearing loss are summarized in Table 6.

Conductive Hearing Loss

Conductive hearing loss results from lesions involving the external or the middle ear. The tympanic membrane and ossicles act as a transformer, amplifying airborne sound and efficiently transferring it to the inner ear fluid. If this normal pathway is obstructed, transmission can occur across the skin and through the bones of the skull (bone conduction) but at the cost of significant energy

---

Table 6 **Features in History That Help Distinguish between Different Types of Hearing Loss**

	Conductive	Sensorineural	Central
Helped by loud speech	yes	no	no
Helped by quiet background	no	yes	yes
Often unilateral	yes	yes	no
Affects certain frequencies only	no	yes	no

Common causes of conductive hearing loss include impacted cerumen and otitis media.

loss. Patients with a conductive hearing loss can hear speech in a noisy background better than in a quiet background, since they can understand loud speech as well as anyone.

The most common cause of conductive hearing loss is impacted cerumen in the external canal. This benign condition is often first noticed after bathing or swimming, when a droplet of water closes the remaining tiny passageway. The most common serious cause of conductive hearing loss is inflammation of the middle ear, otitis media.[1] Either infected fluid (from suppurative otitis) or noninfected fluid (from serous otitis) accumulates in the middle ear, impairing the conduction of airborne sound. With chronic otitis media, a cholesteatoma may erode the ossicles. Otosclerosis produces progressive conductive hearing loss by immobilizing the stapes with new bone growth in front of and below the oval window. Other common causes of conductive hearing loss are trauma, congenital malformations of the external and the middle ear, and glomus body tumors.

Sensorineural Hearing Loss

Sensorineural hearing loss results from lesions of the cochlea, the auditory division of the acoustic nerve (cranial nerve VIII), or both. The spiral cochlea mechanically analyzes the frequency content of sound. For high-frequency tones, only sensory cells in the basilar turn are activated, but for low-frequency tones, all (or nearly all) sensory cells are activated. Therefore, with lesions of the cochlea and its afferent nerve, the hearing levels for different frequencies are usually unequal and the phase relationship (timing) between different frequencies may be altered. Patients with sensorineural hearing loss often have difficulty hearing speech that is mixed with background noise, and they may be annoyed by loud speech.

Distortion of sounds is common with sensorineural hearing loss. A pure tone may be heard as noisy, rough, or buzzing, or it may be distorted so that it sounds like a complex mixture of tones. **Binaural diplacusis** occurs when the two ears are affected unequally, so that the same frequency has a different pitch in each ear (i.e., the patient hears double). **Monaural diplacusis** occurs when two tones, or a tone and a noise, are heard simultaneously in one ear. With **recruitment** there is an abnormally rapid growth in the sensation of loudness as the intensity of a sound is increased; faint or moderate sounds cannot be heard, but there is little or no change in the loudness of loud sounds.

The most common cause of sudden unilateral sensorineural hearing loss is infection of the inner ear (**labyrinthitis**).[2] Bacteria can enter the inner ear directly from the middle ear as a result of recurrent or chronic otitis media or from the CSF via the cochlear aqueduct and internal auditory canal in a patient who has bacterial meningitis. Viral neurolabyrinthitis may be part of a systemic viral illness, such as measles, mumps, or infectious mononucleosis, or an isolated infection of the labyrinth or eighth nerve may occur without systemic symptoms. Mumps is a particularly common cause of unilateral hearing loss in preschool- and school-aged children. Other common causes of acute unilateral hearing loss are head trauma and vascular occlusive disease.

Relapsing unilateral sensorineural hearing loss associated with tinnitus, ear fullness, and vertigo is typical of Ménière's disease. Acoustic neuromas (vestibular schwannomas) characteristically produce a slowly progressive unilateral sensorineural hearing loss.

Ototoxic drugs produce a bilateral subacute hearing loss. The chronic progressive bilateral hearing loss associated with advancing age is called **presbycusis**. It may include conductive and central dysfunction, but the most consistent effect of aging is on the sensory cells and neurons of the cochlea.

> *Sudden unilateral sensorineural hearing loss often is the result of infection.*

> *The progressive bilateral hearing loss associated with aging is primarily sensorineural.*

Central Hearing Loss

Central hearing loss results from lesions of the central auditory pathways. As described in Chapter 4, these lesions involve the cochlear and dorsal olivary nuclear complexes, inferior colliculi, medial geniculate bodies, auditory cortex in the temporal lobes, and interconnecting afferent and efferent fiber tracts. As a rule, patients with central lesions do not have impaired hearing levels for pure tones, and they understand speech as long as it is clearly spoken in a quiet environment. If the listener's task is made more difficult with the introduction of background or competing messages, performance deteriorates more markedly in patients with central lesions than it does in normal subjects (see Central Auditory Speech Tests, later in this chapter). Lesions involving the eighth nerve root entry zone or cochlear nucleus (e.g., demyelination or infarction in the lateral pontomedullary region), however, can cause unilateral hearing loss for pure tones. Because about half of afferent nerve fibers cross central to the cochlear nucleus, this is the most central structure in which a lesion can result in a unilateral hearing loss.

OTOSCOPY

Normal and Abnormal Findings

Otoscopy is performed with the largest speculum that fits comfortably into the external ear canal; to straighten the canal, the pinna is gently pulled posteriorly and superiorly.[3] The tympanic membrane is normally translucent; changes in color indicate middle ear disease (e.g., an amber color suggests a middle ear effusion). **Tympanosclerosis**, a consequence of resolving otitis media or trauma, appears as a semicircular crescent or horseshoe-shaped white plaque within the tympanic membrane. It is rarely associated with hearing loss but is an important clue to past otitic infections. The pars flaccida region (the area superior to the lateral process of the malleus) should be carefully inspected for evidence of a retraction pocket or attic cholesteatoma (see Fig. 3). The ossicles and the color of the underlying mucous membrane of the middle ear can often be assessed through a normally translucent tympanic membrane. **Pneumatoscopy** allows one to determine the mobility of the tympanic membrane. Lack of mobility may indicate an unsuspected perforation, fluid in the middle ear, or severe scarring of the tympanic membrane or middle ear.

Fistula Test

Pressure changes in the ear canal cause nystagmus or slow ocular deviation in patients with a variety of inner ear disorders.

A **fistula test** is performed by transiently changing the pressure in the external ear canal with a pneumatoscope or by pressing the tragus into the canal. A positive fistula sign occurs when there is a transient burst of nystagmus and vertigo.[4] The resulting nystagmus usually lasts from 10 to 20 seconds. The direction of the nystagmus may be either toward or away from the involved ear and is often the same for both positive and negative pressure changes. A positive test indicates a communication between the middle and the inner ear. It usually occurs in patients with a perforated tympanic membrane or erosion of the bony labyrinth due to chronic infection, surgery, or trauma.

Hennebert's sign is a slow ocular deviation (toward or away from the affected ear) after pressure changes in the ear canal that may be followed by at most a few beats of nystagmus, even with sustained pressure. It has been reported in patients with Ménière's disease; congenital syphilis; and ruptures of the oval window, the round window, or both. Hennebert's sign, however, can occasionally be elicited during routine pneumatoscopy in normal subjects, usually bilaterally.

BEDSIDE TESTS OF HEARING

A rough assessment of hearing levels can be performed with very little equipment.

A quick test for hearing loss in the speech range is to observe the response to spoken commands at different intensities (whisper, conversation, shouting). The examiner stands behind the patient to prevent lip reading and occludes and masks the nontest ear by moving a finger back and forth in the patient's external ear canal. A high-frequency stimulus such as a finger snap or coin click (approximately 4000 Hz) may also be used since sensorineural disorders often involve only the higher frequencies.

Tuning fork tests permit a rough assessment of the hearing level for pure tones of known frequency.[3] The examiner's own hearing level can be used as a reference standard. The **Rinne test** compares the patient's hearing by air conduction with that by bone conduction. The fork (preferably 512 Hz) is first held against the mastoid process until the sound fades. It is then placed 1 inch from the ear. Normal subjects can hear the fork about twice as long by air as by bone conduction. If bone conduction is greater than air conduction, a conductive hearing loss is suggested. The **Weber test** compares the patient's hearing by bone conduction in the two ears. The fork is placed at the center of the forehead or on a central incisor, and the patient is asked where he or she hears the tone. Normal subjects hear it in the center of the head, patients with unilateral conductive loss hear it on the affected side, and patients with unilateral sensorineural loss hear it on the side opposite the loss.

STANDARD AUDIOMETRY

Audiometry typically consists of a battery of tests, the differential results of which provide site-of-lesion information.[5]

Pure Tone Studies

Pure tones are defined by their frequency and intensity. To quantify the magnitude of hearing loss, normal hearing levels for pure tones are defined by an international standard. These levels approximate the intensity of the faintest sound that can be heard by normal ears. A patient's hearing level is the difference in decibels (dB) between the faintest pure tone that the patient can hear and the normal reference level given by the standard. Brief-duration pure tones at selected frequencies are presented via earphones (to test air conduction) and via a vibrator pressed against the mastoid portion of the temporal bone (bone conduction). The results of air and bone conduction testing are plotted on an audiogram from which the magnitude (in dB) and configuration (sensitivity loss as a function of frequency) of the hearing loss can be determined (Fig. 38).

With conductive hearing loss, air conduction is impaired but bone conduction remains normal (producing an air–bone gap on the audiogram, as in Fig. 38). Measurement of bone conduction requires careful masking of the nontest ear, since a failure to use masking may result in a false impression of inner ear function. Masking involves introducing a noise into the nontest ear to eliminate inaccurate threshold levels that result from cross-hearing.

Masking of the nontest ear is especially important when testing bone conduction.

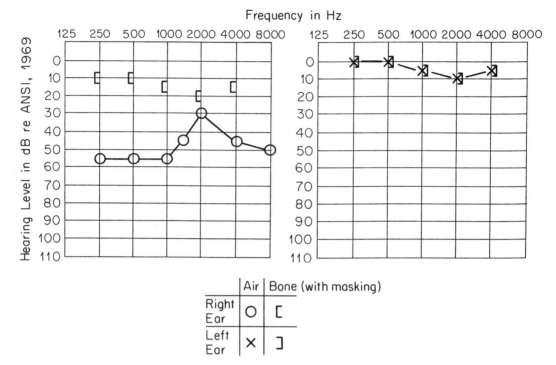

FIGURE 38   Pure tone audiogram: left ear is normal; right ear shows conductive hearing loss due to otosclerosis.

For a bone conduction receiver placed on any part of the skull, the attenuation between the two ears is less than 5 dB.[6] Therefore, a nonhearing ear may appear to have near-normal hearing via bone conduction if the normal ear is not properly masked. The best masking sound for pure tones is a narrow band of white noise centered about the pure tone being tested.

Lesions producing sensorineural hearing loss impair both air and bone conduction, often with changing pure tone levels at different frequencies. Typical audiogram pure tone patterns seen in patients with four common causes of sensorineural hearing loss are shown in Figure 39. None of these patterns is pathognomonic of a given disorder, but they occur often enough to be of diagnostic use.

Some common causes of sensorineural hearing loss tend to produce typical patterns on the pure tone audiogram.

Speech Studies

Two types of tests are used to determine the patient's ability to hear and understand speech. The **speech reception threshold (SRT)** is the intensity at which the patient can correctly repeat 50% of highly familiar two-syllable words (e.g., airplane, cowboy, or sidewalk). The SRT is an estimate of the minimum level of conversation that a person can hear. It provides a check on the validity of the pure tone tests, since it should agree with an average of the two best pure tone thresholds on the audiogram (± 5

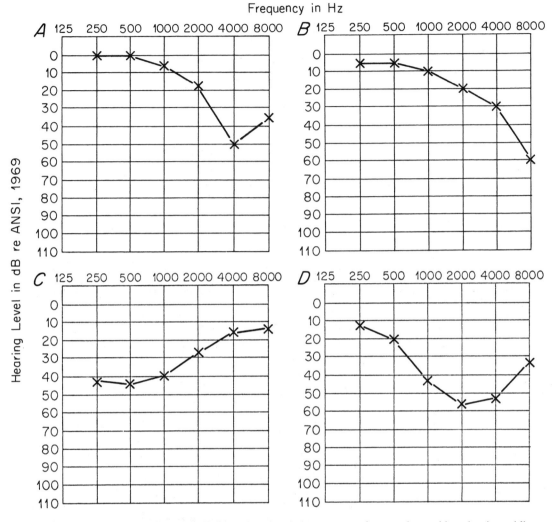

Frequency in Hz

FIGURE 39 Audiograms illustrating four characteristic patterns of sensorineural hearing loss. (A) Notched pattern of noise-induced hearing loss; (B) downward-sloping pattern of presbycusis; (C) low-frequency trough of Ménière's syndrome; and (D) V-pattern of congenital hearing loss.

dB). It is not a test of discrimination, but it does provide information about a patient's ability to recognize and respond to speech.

The **speech discrimination test** is a measure of the patient's ability to understand speech when it is presented at a level that is easily heard. For this test the patient is usually presented with 50 phonetically balanced monosyllabic words at a comfortable listening level. Each word is presented with a carrier phrase such as "You will say ___" or "Say the word ___." The test is scored as a percentage of correct responses, such as 49 out of 50 correct = 98% speech discrimination. In patients with eighth-nerve lesions, speech discrimination can be severely reduced even when pure tone thresholds are normal or near normal. In patients with cochlear lesions, on the other hand, discrimination tends to be proportional to the magnitude of hearing loss.[7]

Recruitment

The **alternate binaural loudness balance (ABLB) test** provides a direct measurement of loudness recruitment if the hearing loss is unilateral. A short-duration tone is presented alternately to each ear. The intensity of the tone to one ear is fixed, while the intensity to the other ear is adjusted until the listener perceives the loudness of the two tones to be equal. Recruitment of loudness is present if the patient requires a smaller-intensity increase (above threshold in quiet) in the hearing-impaired ear than is required in the better-hearing ear to achieve equal loudness between the two ears. Recruitment is typically seen with lesions involving the cochlea.

Tone Decay

Lesions involving the auditory nerve often produce abnormal tone decay.

Tone decay can be measured using a continuously variable or automatic (Bekesy-type) audiometer.[5] In either case, a stimulus is presented continuously at the starting intensity level, and the examiner records the length of time the stimulus is audible to the patient. Under the manual presentation method, the examiner increases the intensity of the signal until the patient can perceive the tone for 60 seconds at a constant intensity level. Using the Bekesy audiometer, a graphic representation of the intensity level required for the patient to maintain audibility of the tone is obtained. Abnormal tone decay is typically seen with lesions involving the auditory nerve.

IMPEDANCE AUDIOMETRY

Impedance may be defined as the resistance of a given system to the flow of energy. **Acoustic impedance** refers to the resistance of the middle ear system to the passage of sound. Its reciprocal, **acoustic compliance**, refers to the ease of sound transmission through the middle ear system. In simplified terms, acoustic impedance indicates the stiffness of the middle ear conduction system; acoustic compliance describes its mobility or springiness. Measurement of acoustic impedance is based on the principle that the **sound pressure level (SPL)** varies with the volume of a closed cavity such as the external ear canal.[8] For a given tone of known frequency and intensity, the SPL decreases as cavity size increases. By measuring the difference between the intensity of a sound going into the external auditory canal and that reflected back from the tympanic membrane, one can estimate the stiffness (or compliance) of the middle ear system.

Acoustic impedance measurements are made via a probe tip hermetically inserted into the ear canal. The probe tip contains three openings: (1) one for air pressure generation and measurement; (2) one for probe tone generation; and (3) one for pickup of sound waves reflected off the tympanic membrane (Fig. 40). With

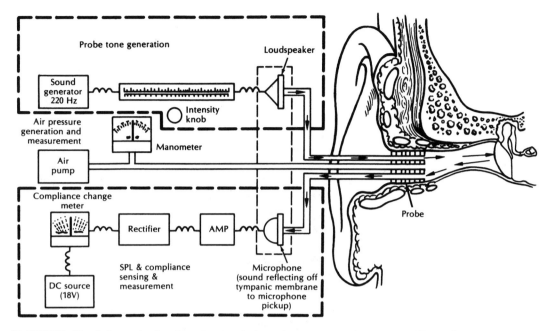

FIGURE 40 Schematic drawing of acoustic impedance measuring system. (From Goodhill, V: *Ear Diseases, Deafness and Dizziness.* Harper & Row, Hagerstown, MD, 1979, p. 188, with permission.)

this system, the difference between generated and reflected sound is systematically measured at different external ear pressure levels.

Static Measurements

A normal middle ear and tympanic membrane offer relatively low acoustic impedance, implying that appreciable energy is absorbed and transmitted through the middle ear. If the middle ear contains fluid or if the tympanic membrane is sclerotic, the acoustic impedance is increased and the transmission capability is diminished; that is, the static compliance is decreased. An increase in acoustic impedance can also result from a decrease in flexibility of the ossicular chain or an increase in its mass or from an increase in friction during ossicular movement. An ossicular chain discontinuity decreases acoustic impedance, since the mass and friction decrease. Unfortunately, acoustic impedance and static compliance measurements rarely provide critical diagnostic information, since the range of normal values is large and values for different otological disorders overlap.

Tympanometry

Tympanometry is a method for evaluating changes in acoustic impedance by producing systematic changes in air pressure in the external ear canal. A plot of compliance change versus air pressure (**tympanogram**) is made by first introducing a positive pressure into the external canal (usually equivalent to $+200$ mm H_2O) and then decreasing the pressure to approximately -200 mm H_2O (although the negative range can be extended to -600 mm H_2O). As the pressure is changed, compliance will change if the conduction system is normal. The shape of a normal tympanogram resembles a teepee (Fig. 41). The peak of the teepee represents the point of maximum compliance, where the air pressure in the middle ear equals the air pressure in the external auditory canal. Tympanometry can provide useful information about mobility of the tympanic membrane, perforations of the tympanic membrane, pressure within the middle ear, and patency and dynamic function of the eustachian tubes.

Abnormal tympanographic patterns suggest various disorders affecting the eardrum and middle ear.

As shown in Figure 41, four characteristic abnormal tympanographic patterns can be identified.[9,10] A restricted tympanogram implies normal middle ear pressure and limited compliance relative to normal mobility. It is typically seen in advanced cases of otosclerosis, lateral fixation of the ossicular chain, tympanic membrane fibrosis, and middle ear tympanosclerosis. A hypermobile tympanogram indicates a flaccid tympanic membrane. It occurs

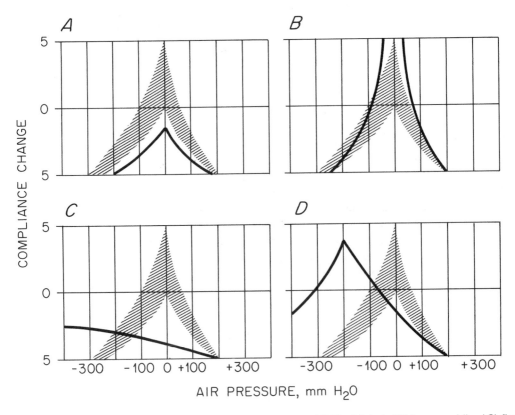

FIGURE 41 Four characteristic abnormal tympanograms. (*A*) Restricted, (*B*) hypermobile, (*C*) flat, and (*D*) retracted. Striped area = normal range.

with ossicular chain discontinuity and with partial atrophy of the tympanic membrane. A flat tympanogram means that there is little or no change in middle ear compliance when air pressure is varied in the external ear canal. This pattern is most commonly seen with serous otitis media but can also be seen with congenital malformations of the middle ear and occlusion of the external ear canal by cerumen, epithelium, and foreign bodies. Finally, with a retracted tympanogram the maximum compliance occurs at negative pressures greater than -100 mm H_2O. It implies a negative middle ear pressure with a retracted tympanic membrane. This pattern is most commonly seen with poor eustachian tube function.

The Acoustic Reflex

The **acoustic reflex** refers to contraction of the stapedius muscle in response to a loud sound (see Fig. 22). It is measured by monitoring the change in acoustic impedance in response to a loud sound introduced into either ear. The stapedius muscle contracts bilaterally, regardless of which ear is stimulated. Contraction of the stapedius muscle produces stiffening of the tympanic membrane and thus an increase in acoustic impedance, which attenuates the sound transmitted to the cochlea by about 10 dB. In a normal subject, the acoustic reflex will be observed when a pure tone signal is presented at 70 to 100 dB above hearing level (median value 82 dB) or when a white noise stimulus is presented at 65 dB above hearing level.[11] By systematically presenting the stimulus sound to each ear and recording with the probe tip in each ear, the location of a lesion within the reflex pathway can be isolated. The results of acoustic reflex testing in patients with four different common unilateral lesions are summarized in Table 7.

Patients with conductive hearing loss often have an absent reflex because the lesion prevents a change in compliance with stapedius muscle contraction. An air–bone gap as small as 5 dB may obscure the acoustic reflex.[12] The acoustic reflex is particularly useful for identifying the site of lesion for different types of

An absent or abnormal acoustic reflex can be used to identify the site of a lesion producing sensorineural hearing loss.

Table 7   **Pattern of Acoustic Reflex Measurements with Unilateral Lesions**

Stimulus Presented:	C	I	C	I
Reflex Measured:	I	C	C	I
Type of Lesion				
Cochlear (<85 dB HL)	+	+	+	+
Conductive (>30 dB HL)	−	−	+	−
Eighth nerve	+	−	+	−
Seventh nerve	−	+	+	−

C = contralateral to lesion; I = ipsilateral to lesion.
+ = reflex present; − = reflex absent.

sensorineural hearing loss. With cochlear lesions, the acoustic reflex often can be demonstrated at a sensation level less than 60 dB above the auditory pure tone threshold. This is another form of abnormal loudness growth or recruitment. A cochlear hearing loss must be severe before the acoustic reflex is lost. An absent reflex is rarely associated with a cochlear hearing loss less than 50 dB, and only when the hearing loss exceeds 85 dB is the reflex absent in 50% of patients.[13] By contrast, patients with eighth-nerve lesions often have either normal or only mildly impaired hearing (less than 20 dB) yet have an abnormal acoustic reflex. The reflex may be absent, exhibit an elevated threshold, or exhibit abnormal decay. Reflex decay is present if the amplitude decreases to one half its original size within 10 seconds of tonal stimulation. The acoustic reflex is abnormal in about 80% of patients with surgically documented acoustic neuromas.[14]

AUDITORY EVOKED RESPONSES

The advent of averaging computers has made it possible to collect and analyze a variety of evoked electrical potentials from the auditory nervous system.[15] Disk electrodes are attached to the head, repetitive sounds are delivered to the external ear, and an "averaged" series of specific brain wave potentials for up to 500 ms after signal onset can be recorded. The latencies (re: signal onset) of each of the brain wave potentials are used as the most reliable means by which generator sources for the potentials in the central nervous system are identified. Specifically, the early (0 to 10 ms) evoked responses reflect the far-field representation of electrical events generated at points from the periphery (nerve VIII action potential) to the level of the brain stem. The five to seven waves in the first 10 ms are referred to as the **brain stem evoked response**. The middle latency responses (12 to 50 ms) have received less systematic study but probably reflect electrical activity in the upper brain stem and in the primary and nearby secondary auditory projection areas. The late evoked responses (50 to 300 ms) reflect cortical electrical activity.

The BAER can test auditory pathways in patients who are unable to cooperate with subjective auditory testing.

The **brain stem auditory evoked response (BAER)** is highly reproducible in a given subject and shows little variation among normal subjects. With rare exceptions the BAER is not affected by inattention to the stimulus, alterations in the level of consciousness, or drugs. For this reason it can be used to test the integrity of the peripheral and brain stem auditory pathways in patients who cannot cooperate with subjective auditory testing (e.g., infants or comatose patients).

A schematic drawing of a BAER and the neuronal centers that are thought to generate each component of the response is shown in Figure 42. Wave I (average latency 1.9 ms) results from activation of the eighth-nerve terminals within the cochlea, while the remainder of the waves are generated by the retrocochlear part of the eighth nerve and the brain stem auditory nuclei and pathways.[16–18] Although a useful working tool, this schematic

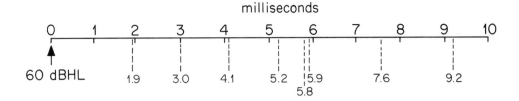

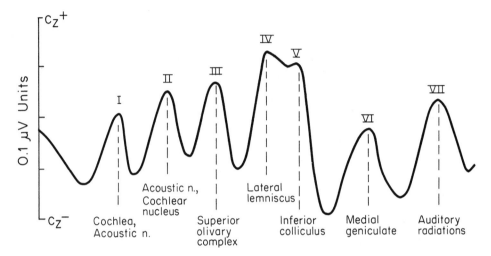

FIGURE 42   Normal brain stem auditory response evoked by clicks of 60 dB HL (60 dB above normal hearing threshold) at a rate of 10 per second. Normal mean latencies for waves I through VII are shown on the time scale (the intermediate latency, 5.8 ms, between waves IV and V, is the mean peak latency of a fused wave IV-V when present). The neural centers thought to be responsible for generating each wave are shown at the bottom. (Adapted from Stockard, JJ, Stockard, JE, and Sharbrough, FW: Detection and localization of occult lesions with brain stem auditory responses. Mayo Clinic Proc 52:761, 1977.)

electroanatomical correlation is an oversimplification. Clearly each vertex-positive and vertex-negative potential after wave I reflects simultaneous activity in multiple brain stem loci. The more caudal generators, such as the eighth nerve, cochlear nuclei, and superior olivary complex, contribute to the response beyond waves II and III. By the time waves VI and VII appear, the summation of potentials from the different neuronal centers is so complex that the concept of single principal contributors to individual waves no longer applies. Therefore, the greatest diagnostic value of BAER is to establish the presence of a central lesion rather than to define its precise location.

The standard stimulus for eliciting BAERs is a click caused by a very short DC pulse. This is a spectrally diffused acoustic stimulus with most of the energy concentrated in the high frequencies (2000 Hz). The absolute latency of the BAER waves is dependent on the intensity of the click stimulus. The BAERs to unfiltered clicks presented at various intensity levels from a normal subject are shown in Figure 43. Wave V is most robust, often being identifiable at only 10 dB above hearing level. At 70 dB above hearing level, all waves are identifiable. Such latency-intensity functions provide a basis for estimating the degree of hearing loss in

The BAER is better at establishing the presence of a central lesion than it is at defining its precise location.

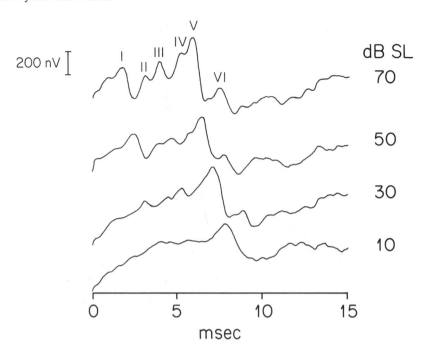

200 nV

dB SL

70

50

30

10

0   5   10   15

msec

FIGURE 43 Brain stem auditory evoked responses in a normal subject induced by clicks at varying intensity levels (10 to 70 dB SL, sensation level).

patients who cannot cooperate with standard pure tone testing.[19,20] On the other hand, because of this latency-intensity relationship, BAERs must be interpreted with caution in patients with severe conductive or cochlear hearing loss (particularly if it involves the high frequencies).

In practice, only waves I, III, and V are used to define response abnormalities. Waves II, IV, VI, and VII are sufficiently variable in the normal population to preclude their routine use in defining response abnormalities on the basis of a single recording. Often waves IV and V fuse into a single complex, which is designated as wave IV/V. Since wave I disappears before wave IV/V with decreasing stimulus intensity (e.g., see Fig. 43), the absence of wave IV/V in the presence of wave I indicates a lesion of the eighth nerve. The absence of all waves, on the other hand, often reflects a peripheral lesion (conductive or cochlear) or a technical problem.[17,21] If peak I occurs at normal latency, then prolongation of the I–III or I–IV/V interval indicates a lesion of the eighth nerve or brain stem.

BAER measurements have been particularly useful for early detection of acoustic neuromas. Abnormal BAERs occur in approximately 95% of surgically proven cases.[22,23] The most common abnormality overall is absence of all waves beyond wave I. For small tumors with minimal or no detectable pure tone hearing loss, prolongation of the I–IV/V interval is the most common finding (Fig. 44).

Electrocochleography is a modification of the brain stem auditory evoked response test in which wave I is amplified to reveal

BAERs are especially useful for early detection of acoustic neuromas.

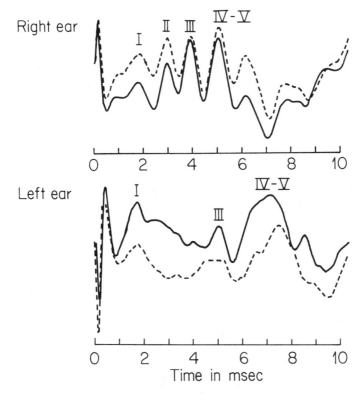

FIGURE 44 Brain stem auditory evoked responses in a patient with a left acoustic neuroma. Dashed lines indicate repeat test. Wave I occurs at normal latency on both sides, but the I–III and I–V intervals are prolonged on the left side.

both the action potential of the cochlear nerve and another wave preceding the action potential, referred to as the **summating potential**.[24] Normally the ratio of the summating potential (SP) to the action potential (AP) is less than 0.4. With Ménière's disease, the SP increases relative to the AP.[25] When the ratio exceeds 0.5, it is abnormal and indicative of Ménière's disease. With early Ménière's disease, however, electrocochleography may show a normal SP/AP ratio. Sometimes repeating electrocochleography when the patient is symptomatic will identify the characteristic change in the SP/AP ratio.

Abnormal results on electrocochleography may indicate Ménière's disease.

CENTRAL AUDITORY SPEECH TESTS

Patients with lesions of the central auditory pathways usually have pure tone thresholds within the normal range. Routine speech tests are also usually normal since speech contains a great deal of redundancy. Within the central auditory pathways, redundancy is enhanced by the multiple crossings and interactions. One of the few diagnostically useful clinical audiological findings is the reduced ability of patients with temporal lobe lesions to discriminate speech in the ear contralateral to the lesion when the task is complicated by distorting the speech.[26] Apparently by making the speech less redundant, heavier demands are placed on the integrating and synthesizing function of the auditory cortex.

Several varieties of central auditory speech tests are currently in use, most involving different methods of presenting distorted speech.[5,26] Portions of the frequency spectrum of speech can be filtered, the speech can be time compressed, it can be presented at very low intensities, and it can be interrupted at irregular intervals. Dichotic stimulation involves presenting two different messages to each ear. Both monosyllabic words and words with two equally stressed syllables can be used. With these tests, when a temporal lobe lesion exists, the ear contralateral to the lesion performs more poorly than the ear ipsilateral to the lesion.

References

1. Brookhouser PE: Sensorineural hearing loss in children. In Cummings CW, et al. (eds): Otolaryngology—Head and Neck Clinic, vol. 4, ed 2. Mosby Year Book, St. Louis, 1993.
2. Wilson WR, and Gulya AJ: Sudden sensorineural hearing loss. In Cummings CW, et al. (eds): Otolaryngology—Head and Neck Clinic, vol. 4, ed 2. Mosby Year Book, St. Louis, 1993.
3. House JW: Otologic and neurotologic history and physical examination. In Cummings CW, et al. (eds): Otolaryngology—Head and Neck Surgery, vol. 4. Mosby Year Book, St. Louis, 1993.
4. Wall C III, and Rauch SD: Perilymphatic fistula. In Baloh RW, and Halmagyi GM (eds): Disorders of the Vestibular System. Oxford University Press, New York, 1996.
5. Rintlemann WF (ed): Hearing Assessment. Perspectives in Audiology Series. PRO-ED, Austin TX, 1991.
6. Heffernan HP, Simons MR, and Goodhill V: Audiologic assessment, functional hearing loss and objective audiometry. In Goodhill V (ed): Ear Diseases, Deafness and Dizziness. Harper & Row, Hagerstown MD, 1979.
7. Jerger J, and Jerger S: Diagnostic significance of PB word functions. Arch Otolaryngol 93:573, 1971.
8. Sheehy JL, and Hughes RL: The ABC's of impedance audiometry. Laryngoscope 84:1935, 1974.
9. Liden G, Pederson GL, and Bjorkman G: Tympanometry. Arch Otolaryngol 92:248, 1970.
10. Jerger J: Clinical experience with impedance audiometry. Arch Otolaryngol 92:311, 1970.
11. Jepson O: Middle ear reflexes in man. In Jerger J (ed): Modern Developments in Audiology. Academic Press, New York, 1963.
12. Jerger J, Anthon L, Jerger S, et al.: Studies in impedance audiometry. III. Middle ear disorders. Arch Otolaryngol 99:165, 1974.
13. Jerger J, Jerger S, and Maulden L: Studies in impedance audiometry. I. Normal and S-N ears. Arch Otolaryngol 96:513, 1972.
14. Sheehy JL, and Inzer BE: Acoustic reflex test in neurotologic diagnosis. Arch Otolaryngol 102:647, 1976.
15. Moller AR: Auditory neurophysiology. J Clin Neurophysiol 11:284, 1994.
16. Starr A, and Hamilton AE: Correlation between confirmed sites of neurological lesions and abnormalities of far-field auditory brainstem responses. Electroencephalogr Clin Neurophysiol 41:595, 1976.
17. Stockard JJ, Stockard JE, and Sharbrough FW: Detection and localization of occult lesions with brainstem auditory responses. Mayo Clin Proc 52:761, 1977.
18. Moller AR, Janetta PJ, and Moller MB: Neural generators of brainstem evoked potentials. Results from human intracranial recordings. Ann Otol Rhinol Laryngol 90:591, 1981.
19. Don M, Eggermont JJ, and Brachmann DE: Reconstruction of the audiogram using brain stem responses and high-pass noise masking. Ann Otol Rhinol Laryngol 88 (Suppl 57):1, 1979.
20. Davis H: Auditory evoked potentials as a method for assessing hearing impairment. Trends Neurosci June 1981:126.

21. Coats AC: Human auditory nerve action potential and brain stem evoked responses. Arch Otolaryngol 104:799, 1978.
22. Josey AF, Jackson GG, and Glasscock ME: Brainstem evoked response audiometry in confirmed eighth nerve tumors. Am J Otolaryngol 1:185, 1980.
23. Wilson DF, Hodgson RS, Gustafson MF, et al.: The sensitivity of auditory brainstem response testing in small acoustic neuromas. Laryngoscope 102:961, 1992.
24. Portmann M: Electrocochleography. J Laryngol 91:665, 1977.
25. Ferraro J, Arenberg IK, and Hassanian RS: Electrocochleography and symptoms of inner ear dysfunction. Arch Otolaryngol 111:71, 1985.
26. Berlin C, Love-Bell S, Janetta P, and Kline D: Central auditory deficits after temporal lobectomy. Arch Otolaryngol 96:4, 1972.

8

Approach to the Patient with Dizziness

Chapter Outline

Because dizziness can represent many different overlapping sensations and can be caused by different pathophysiological mechanisms, it is critical that the examining physician take a careful history to determine the type of dizziness before proceeding with the diagnostic evaluation. The history provides direction for both the examination and the diagnostic workup (Table 8). Although the vestibular system is the focus of this book, many patients complaining of dizziness do not have a disorder of the vestibular system. The clinician should begin by formulating a clinical profile by asking the patient to describe the sensation itself, how it began, how long it lasts, how frequently it occurs, and whether there are circumstances that induce it.[1,2]

Many "dizzy" patients do not have vestibular disorders.

Table 8   Mechanism and Focus of Diagnostic Workup for Different Types of Dizziness

Type of Dizziness	Mechanism	Focus of Evaluation
Vertigo	Imbalance in tonic vestibular signals	Auditory and vestibular systems
Near-faint dizziness	Decreased blood flow to the entire brain	Cardiovascular system
Psychophysiological dizziness	Impaired central integration of sensory signals	Psychiatric assessment
Hypoglycemic dizziness	Inadequate brain glucose; increased circulatory catecholamines	Metabolic assessment
Disequilibrium	Loss of sensorimotor control	Peripheral nerves, spinal cord, inner ear, vision, central nervous system

DISTINGUISHING BETWEEN DIFFERENT TYPES OF DIZZINESS

Vertigo

Events just prior to an episode of dizziness are important in determining the cause. Dizziness caused by vestibular lesions is usually worsened by rapid head movements since the new stimulus is sensed by the intact labyrinth and existing asymmetries are accentuated. Episodes of vertigo (described in Chapter 5) may be precipitated by turning over in bed, sitting up from the lying position, extending the neck to look up, or bending over and straightening up. Patients with a perilymph fistula have brief episodes of vertigo precipitated by changes in middle ear pressure (coughing, sneezing).[3] The pressure change in the middle ear is transferred directly to the inner ear (usually the horizontal semicircular canal) (see Fig. 76). Occasionally, loud noises induce transient vertigo in patients with Ménière's disease (**Tulio phenomenon**). As the labyrinthine membranes dilate because of increased endolymphatic pressure, adhesions may develop between the stapedius footplate and the membranous labyrinth, resulting in traction on the sensory receptors with sudden movement of the stapes (see Fig. 71).[4]

The nervous system has a remarkable ability to compensate for an imbalance within the vestibular system, and thus dizziness due to vestibular lesions usually occurs in episodes. Of the commonly encountered vestibular syndromes, brief episodes lasting only seconds are typical of benign paroxysmal positional vertigo. Episodes lasting minutes are characteristic of vascular syndromes, such as transient vertebrobasilar insufficiency and migraine. Vertigo during a typical bout of Ménière's disease lasts for 3 to 4 hours, although the patient often complains of a vague

Episodic vertigo is typical of peripheral vestibular disorders.

sense of dizziness for a day or so thereafter. Viral labyrinthitis and mononeuritis of the vestibular nerve (vestibular neuritis) are characterized by the acute onset of severe vertigo followed by gradually decreasing intensity over several days. Continuous dizziness without fluctuation for long periods of time is not typical of peripheral vestibular disorders.

The severity of symptoms following a vestibular lesion depends on the extent of the lesion, whether it is unilateral or bilateral, and the rapidity with which the functional loss occurs. Patients who slowly lose vestibular function bilaterally (e.g., secondary to ototoxic drugs) often do not complain of dizziness but will report oscillopsia with head movements, due to loss of vestibulo-ocular reflex activity, and instability when walking, from loss of vestibulospinal reflex activity. If a patient slowly loses vestibular function on one side only over a period of months to years (e.g., with an acoustic neuroma), symptoms and signs may be absent. On the other hand, a sudden unilateral loss of vestibular function is a dramatic event. The patient complains of severe vertigo and nausea and is pale and perspiring and usually vomits repeatedly. Such patients prefer to lie quietly in a dark room but can walk if forced to (falling toward the side of the lesion). A brisk, spontaneous nystagmus interferes with vision. These symptoms and signs are transient, and the process of compensation begins almost immediately. Within 1 week of the lesion, a young patient can walk without difficulty and, with fixation, can inhibit the spontaneous nystagmus. Within a month, most patients return to work with few, if any, residual symptoms.

Unfortunately, the description of vertigo does not differentiate peripheral from central lesions. For this, one must rely on the associated symptoms. Lesions of the labyrinth or eighth cranial nerve usually produce auditory symptoms such as hearing loss, tinnitus, a sensation of pressure or fullness in the ear, and pain in the ear. In addition to hearing loss and tinnitus, lesions of the internal auditory canal are often associated with ipsilateral facial weakness. Lesions in the cerebellopontine angle may cause ipsilateral facial numbness and weakness and ipsilateral extremity ataxia.

The association of vertigo with other symptoms may help to localize the lesion.

Because of the close approximation of other neuronal centers and fiber tracts in the brain stem and cerebellum, it is unusual to find lesions in these areas that produce isolated vestibular symptoms. Lesions of the brain stem invariably are associated with other cranial nerve and long-tract symptoms. For example, vertigo caused by transient vertebrobasilar insufficiency is associated with other brain stem and occipital lobe symptoms such as diplopia, hemianoptic field defects, drop attacks, weakness, numbness, dysarthria, and ataxia. Lesions of the cerebellum (e.g., infarction or hemorrhage) may be relatively silent but are always associated with extremity and truncal ataxia in addition to vertigo. Of note, hearing loss for pure tones is unusual with brain stem lesions, even in the late stages.

Vertigo can occur as part of an aura of temporal lobe seizures. The cortical projections of the vestibular system are activated by a focal discharge within the temporal lobe. Such vertigo is nearly always associated with other typical aura symptoms, such as an abnormal taste or smell and distortion of the visual world (hallucinations and illusions). Occasionally, however, vertigo can be the only manifestation of an aura. In such cases the association with typical "absence" spells should lead one to the correct diagnosis.

Near-Faint Dizziness

Near-faint dizziness suggests reduced blood flow to the entire brain.

Near-faint dizziness or **presyncope** refers to the light-headed sensation one experiences before losing consciousness or fainting. It is usually easily distinguished from vertigo because there is no illusion of motion and no associated loss of balance. Conditions producing near-faint dizziness are in large part the same conditions that cause syncope (Table 9).[5,6] The mechanism is reduced blood flow to the entire brain. When cerebral blood flow is partially reduced, patients experience light-headedness; when there is greater reduction, syncope occurs. Consequently, recurrent presyncopal light-headedness often proceeds to syncope at some point. Near-faint dizziness is not a symptom of focal occlusion of the carotid or the vertebrobasilar system.

Orthostatic Hypotension

Orthostatic hypotension is usually due to acute blood loss, volume depletion, and diuretics or antihypertensive medications.[6] Older patients are especially susceptible to these factors. Less often, autonomic dysfunction or central neurogenic causes are responsible. When the patient stands, gravitational pooling of blood occurs in the limbs and splanchnic vasculature. This pooling causes reduced blood pressure, which in turn reduces cerebral perfusion pressure, leading most patients to experience dizziness. The more precipitous the drop in blood pressure in the upright position, the more likely it is to result in syncope.

The diagnosis rests on documenting a decrement greater than 20 mm Hg in systolic blood pressure in the upright position com-

---

Table 9   **Common Causes of Near-Faint Dizziness**

Orthostatic hypotension
    Volume depletion
    Vasodilators, antihypertensive drugs, anaphylaxis, shock
    Autonomic dysfunction
Cardiac disease
    Cardiomyopathy
    Aortic stenosis
    Constrictive pericarditis
    Arrhythmias, conduction defects
Vasovagal presyncope
Hyperventilation

pared with the supine position. The patient should be evaluated for anemia and signs of volume depletion and for signs of autonomic dysfunction most commonly associated with peripheral neuropathy. Treatment is directed at the cause whenever possible.[7] Orthostatic hypotension may respond to thigh or abdominal high compression stockings and increased dietary salt intake.

Cardiac Disease

Cardiovascular causes of near-faint dizziness produce symptoms identical to those of orthostatic hypotension except that they may occur while sitting and occasionally even while lying down. Dizziness associated with exertion, chest pain, palpitations, a heart murmur, or electrocardiogram (ECG) abnormalities should prompt a thorough cardiac evaluation. Cardiac dysrhythmia, cardiomyopathy, constrictive pericarditis, and aortic stenosis are all conditions that reduce cardiac output, causing syncope or near-syncope.

Near-faint dizziness can usually be traced to a cardiovascular cause.

Vasovagal Presyncope

Vasovagal or neurally mediated presyncope is probably the most common cause of presyncope.[5] Like orthostatic hypotension, most episodes occur when the patient is standing, but unlike orthostatic hypotension, the blood pressure is not necessarily reduced immediately upon standing. Initial symptoms include nausea and diaphoresis followed by light-headedness, dimness of vision, and pallor. These symptoms are often situational; that is, they may be associated with hunger, emotional stress, prolonged standing, or exposure to excessive heat or strong odors or may be the result of acute pain or intense vertigo. The mechanism is not fully understood but begins with an afferent signal from arteriovisceral mechanoreceptors. An efferent parasympathetic reflex then may produce bradycardia followed by vasodilatation of capacitance vessels, particularly in the splanchnic vascular bed. In some cases, a vasodepressor phenomenon can occur without the antecedent bradycardia or any other warning. Head-up tilt-table testing can be useful for confirming the diagnosis.

The most common type of presyncope is vasovagal, in which symptoms of near-faint dizziness are often situational and follow other symptoms.

Hyperventilation

Hyperventilation is a common cause of near-faint dizziness in anxious young people.[8] Patients describe light-headedness, giddiness, perioral and acral numbness and tingling, globus hystericus (lump in the throat), deep sighing, and feelings of suffocation and chest pressure. The symptom complex may resemble psychophysiological dizziness as well as near-faint dizziness. Rapid respirations reduce the pCO_2 to the point of cerebral vasoconstriction. If brief periods of voluntary hyperventilation (less than a minute) reproduce the symptoms exactly, the diagnosis is confirmed.

Table 10   **Features of Psychophysiological Dizziness**

Description	Floating, swimming, rocking, giddy, depersonalized, spinning inside the head (environment remains still)
Associated symptoms	Tension headaches, palpitations, gastric distress, urinary frequency, backache, generalized weakness, and fatigue
Common situations that provoke attacks	Walking on a brightly polished floor or down a supermarket aisle, driving on a freeway, shopping in a crowded store, death of a loved one

Psychophysiological Dizziness

The mechanism of psychophysiological dizziness appears to be altered central integration of sensory signals arising from normal end organs.[9] In some cases, it seems as though patients are simply overfocused on normal physiological sensations. In other cases, such as patients with panic syndrome, a neurochemical malady is likely. Most theories focus on inappropriate release of neurotransmitters within the brain, particularly catecholamines. Common features of psychophysiological dizziness are summarized in Table 10.

Anxiety

Dizziness associated with anxiety is usually a vague sensation of floating or giddiness along with fatigue. These patients commonly have symptoms when they are alone, sitting quietly and ruminating about their problem. They may feel separated from their body but rarely lose balance, fall, or become nauseated. Symptoms may be intermittent or may last for years, varying in intensity from day to day. Common causes of anxiety in daily life are circumstances in which one must make a decision that could have major implications for future social and economic status. The symptoms associated with this type of anxiety are usually transitory and completely reversible.[10] Anxiety can also be associated with a number of neurologic and psychiatric disorders. For example, the first sign of dementia or manic-depressive illness can be an attack of severe anxiety without obvious cause.

Panic Syndrome

Chronic dizziness is commonly associated with panic syndrome, a psychiatric disorder with a genetic predisposition.

Panic syndrome is a distinct psychiatric diagnostic category characterized by panic attacks and multiple other symptoms, including chronic dizziness (Table 11).[11] Panic attacks are sudden attacks of fear and impending doom that usually last 10 to 20 minutes. The dizziness can take several forms, from a giddy, unsteady sensation to a progressing near-faint dizziness due to the associated hyperventilation. As typically seen with hyperventila-

Table 11	**Common Symptoms during Panic Attacks**

Shortness of breath, smothering, choking
Palpitations, accelerated heart rate
Chest pain or discomfort
Sweating
Dizziness, unsteady feeling, sensory illusions
Nausea or abdominal distress
Depersonalization or derealization
Numbness or tingling sensations (paresthesias)
Flushes (hot flashes) or chills
Trembling or shaking
Fear of dying
Fear of going crazy or doing something uncontrolled

tion, the patient experiences a tightness in the chest as though the lungs cannot be adequately filled. The patient may try to flee and in the future avoid the situation in which the panic attack occurred. Panic syndrome has a clear genetic predisposition, distinguishing it from the more common anxieties that are responses to specific life situations. Some patients improve with reassurance and self-relaxation. Disabling symptoms may require medical treatment in conjunction with counseling.[12] Tricyclic amines, selective serotonin reuptake inhibitors, and alprazolam are effective medications used in treating panic syndrome and the related dizziness.

Phobic Dizziness

Phobic vertigo or **phobic dizziness** is a morbid fear of falling unassociated with postural or gait instability. It is often associated with panic syndrome and agoraphobia, although patients may focus on the physical symptoms, so that the associated symptoms of anxiety are only uncovered with detailed questioning. Patients have a fear of falling when sitting or standing, and active body movements provoke unpleasant illusions of body acceleration with simultaneous illusory movement of the stationary environment. Often patients will have a sudden desire to flee from the place at which the attack is provoked and, if seated, will rigidly grasp the arm of the chair to avoid falling from the chair. Anticipatory anxiety leads to further attacks of dizziness despite the discrepancy between the subjective fear of falling and the absence of objective unsteadiness. Some of these patients develop agoraphobia, but others are able to continue their social and work habits despite symptoms that they feel are dominating their lives.[13]

Hypoglycemic Dizziness

Hypoglycemia may lead to behavioral changes, light-headedness, lethargy, confusion, amnesia, seizures, weakness, shakiness, fatigue, and diaphoresis. It usually is a complication of insulin or

Dizziness in diabetic patients may result from hypoglycemia.

sulfonylurea treatment in diabetic patients, but it may occur with insulinomas or as a fasting or postprandial phenomenon. Postprandial symptoms of shakiness, palpitations, fatigue, and dizziness have been termed **functional hypoglycemia** because most such cases are not associated with significantly low plasma glucose levels. The history in patients suspected of having hypoglycemia should focus on whether insulin or sulfonylureas have been taken. Diagnosis rests on measuring plasma glucose, insulin, and c-peptide. c-Peptide is the connecting peptide that is cleaved from proinsulin to form insulin.[14] Elevation of c-peptide and insulin suggests excessive endogenous insulin (such as from an insulinoma). An elevated insulin level with normal or suppressed c-peptide level indicates excessive exogenous insulin, since c-peptide is not present in pharmaceutical insulin and is in fact suppressed by it.

Disequilibrium

Patients often use the term "dizziness" to describe a sensation of imbalance or disequilibrium that occurs only when they are standing or walking and is unrelated to an abnormal head sensation. Imbalance is common with acute unilateral peripheral vestibular lesions, but it is transient and invariably associated with subjective vertigo. Both the vertigo and the imbalance are compensated for within a few days. Patients who slowly lose vestibular function on one side, such as with an acoustic neuroma, may not experience vertigo but often describe a vague feeling of imbalance and unsteadiness on their feet. By contrast, bilateral symmetrical vestibular loss causes a more pronounced, persistent unsteadiness that may be incapacitating, particularly in older patients.

Disequilibrium is a particularly common problem in older patients.[15] It is typically described as a feeling of dizziness when standing or walking that is not present while sitting or lying down. It is usually worse upon first standing or when bending over or turning rapidly. The symptoms and associated fear of falling affect the patient's quality of life and may limit daily activities. Falls are a well-known source of morbidity among these older patients. Even after a careful history and examination, the cause for gait imbalance in older people is often unclear.[16] The difficulty of assigning cause may be complicated by the confounding effects of medications, weakness, deconditioning, musculoskeletal limitations, and effort.

The risk of falls increases linearly with age after age 60 and is greater in women than in men.[17,18] Most falls by older people result from an accidental slip or trip. The cause can often be traced to decreased sensory inputs, slowing of responses, and weakness of support. Sedating medications are a common contributing factor. Falls can be directly traced to an acute attack of dizziness in fewer than 10% of patients. This low incidence probably can be attributed to the fact that most types of dizziness, including attacks of vertigo, begin slowly enough to allow the patient to sit down or to grab on to a support to avoid falling.

Considering the many possible loci of dysfunction, examination of a patient complaining of disequilibrium must include a careful assessment of gait, strength, coordination, reflexes, and sensory function, particularly of the lower extremities (see Fig. 49). The broad-based atactic gait of cerebellar disorders and the shuffling apractic gait of subcortical white-matter disease are readily distinguished from the milder gait disorders seen with vestibular or proprioceptive loss. Bilateral vestibular loss may or may not be associated with hearing loss. The diagnosis rests on finding decreased or absent response to caloric and rotational stimulation.

Many factors must be assessed in the examination of the older patient with disequilibrium, a sensation of imbalance when standing or walking without an abnormal head sensation.

Drug-Induced Dizziness

A careful history regarding medications is critical in evaluating any patient complaining of dizziness (Table 12). Ototoxic drugs such as the aminoglycosides and cisplatin can cause vertigo if hair cell loss is asymmetrical, but more often they cause disequilibrium and oscillopsia from bilateral symmetrical end organ damage.[19] Carbamazepine, phenytoin, primidone, and alcohol can cause acute reversible disequilibrium and chronic irreversible disequilibrium from cerebellar dysfunction. Sedating drugs cause a nonspecific dizziness typically described as a fogginess, cloudiness, or giddiness that is presumably due to diffuse depression of the central nervous system. A number of commonly used drugs produce a characteristic drug intoxication syndrome that might be confused with other types of dizziness. The associated confusion, disorientation, memory and cognitive deficits, gaze-evoked nystagmus, and gait and extremity ataxia indicate combined cortical and cerebellar dysfunction.[20] These drugs affect multiple neurotransmitters within the CNS, but the cause of the drug intoxication syndrome is unknown. The most commonly recognized syndrome

Many common drugs produce a syndrome that can easily be confused with other causes of dizziness.

Table 12   Type and Mechanism of Dizziness Associated with Commonly Used Drugs

Drug	Type of Dizziness	Mechanism
Aminoglycosides, cisplatin	Vertigo, disequilibrium	Damage to vestibular hair cells
Antiepileptics: carbamazepine, phenytoin, primidone	Disequilibrium, intoxication	Cerebellar toxicity, CNS depression
Tranquilizers: barbiturates, benzodiazepines, tricyclic amines, marijuana	Intoxication	CNS depression
Antihypertensives, diuretics	Near-faint	Postural hypotension, reduced cerebral blood flow
Alcohol	Intoxication, disequilibrium, positional vertigo	CNS depression, cerebellar toxicity, change in cupula's specific gravity

is that associated with alcohol ingestion. A light-headed, swimming sensation is typically associated with slowing of cognitive functions and motor responses. Gaze-evoked nystagmus with horizontal gaze deviation and gait ataxia are early reliable signs of the syndrome. With increased intoxication, gaze-evoked nystagmus occurs with vertical gaze deviation, and the upper extremities are atactic. The alcohol concentration in the blood can be reasonably well predicted by the degree of gaze-evoked nystagmus.

The diagnosis rests on finding the characteristic combination of symptoms and signs in a patient taking one of the offending drugs. Blood levels can now be routinely obtained on most of these drugs, so a specific diagnosis is possible.

Summary: Vestibular versus Nonvestibular Types of Dizziness

The patient's description, aggravating factors, and associated symptoms all help in distinguishing between vestibular and nonvestibular causes of dizziness.

Although the description alone does not distinguish between vestibular and nonvestibular causes of dizziness, certain words are commonly used to describe each type of dizziness (Table 13). A sensation of spinning nearly always indicates a vestibular disorder. Patients with nonvestibular dizziness occasionally report a sensation of spinning inside the head but the environment remains still, and they do not have nystagmus. Patients with vestibular lesions liken the sensation to that of being drunk or motion sick. They describe feelings of imbalance as though they are falling or tilting to one side. In patients with nonvestibular dizziness, illusions of motion of the environment are rare but illusions of self-movement are common. These patients typically use terms such as light-headed, floating, rocking, giddy, or swimming. The sensation that one has left one's body is characteristic of psychophysiological dizziness.

One must keep in mind, however, that well-documented lesions within the vestibular system sometimes produce only a nonspecific sensation of disorientation without a clearly defined illusion of movement. Normal subjects undergoing caloric stimulation (a physiological imbalance in the vestibular system) occasionally

Table 13 Distinguishing between Vestibular and Nonvestibular Causes of Dizziness

Factor	Vestibular	Nonvestibular
Common descriptive terms	Spinning (environment moves), merry-go-round, drunkenness, tilting, motion sickness, off balance	Light-headed, floating, dissociated from body, swimming, giddy, spinning inside (environment stationary)
Course	Episodic	Constant
Common precipitating or aggravating factors	Head movements, position change	Stress, hyperventilation, cardiac arrhythmias, situations
Commonly associated symptoms	Nausea, vomiting, unsteadiness, tinnitus, hearing loss, impaired vision, oscillopsia	Paresthesias, syncope, difficulty concentrating, tension headache

describe the experience with terms such as floating or even giddiness. For these reasons, dizziness cannot be classified on the basis of subjective description alone.

Vertigo is an episodic phenomenon, whereas nonvestibular dizziness is often continuous, except for presyncopal light-headedness caused by postural hypotension or cardiac arrhythmia. Patients with psychophysiological dizziness often report being dizzy from morning to night without change for months to years at a time. Vertigo is invariably aggravated by head movements, whereas nonvestibular dizziness may even improve with head or body movements. Episodes of dizziness induced by position change suggest a vestibular lesion if postural hypotension has been ruled out. Although stress can aggravate both vestibular and nonvestibular dizziness, dizziness that is reliably precipitated by stress suggests a nonvestibular cause. Finally, episodes of dizziness that occur only in specific situations (e.g., driving on a freeway, entering a crowded room, or shopping in a busy supermarket) suggest a nonvestibular cause.

The presence of associated symptoms also can help one distinguish between vestibular and nonvestibular causes of dizziness. Nausea and vomiting are usual with vertigo but are uncommon with other types of dizziness. Associated auditory or neurologic symptoms suggest a vestibular disorder, whereas presyncopal symptoms and syncope suggest a nonvestibular cause. Multiple symptoms of acute and chronic anxiety commonly accompany psychophysiological dizziness.

WORKUP OF COMMON PRESENTATIONS OF VESTIBULAR DIZZINESS

Acute Prolonged Attack of Vertigo

Acute, spontaneous vertigo results from a sudden unilateral impairment of vestibular function. It can result from sudden loss of peripheral input caused by damage to the labyrinth or vestibular nerve, or it can be caused by a sudden unilateral impairment of vestibular nuclear or vestibulocerebellar activity. The patient experiences an intense sensation of rotation aggravated by head motion and usually made worse by lying down. It is relieved by sitting upright and keeping the head still or by lying with the intact side undermost. There also might be a sense of self-tilting toward the affected side. Because of the spontaneous nystagmus, the patient usually notices that the visual world is moving slowly in one direction and quickly back in the other direction. Standing and walking are difficult and the patient may fall toward the affected side. There are nearly always associated autonomic symptoms, including malaise, pallor, sweating, nausea, vomiting, and sometimes diarrhea. The first task of the examining physician is to determine whether the vertigo is of central or peripheral origin, because some central causes of acute vertigo can be life threatening and may require immediate intervention (Fig. 45).

In examining a patient with acute, prolonged vertigo, the first task is to rule out a possible central cause requiring immediate intervention.

Acute spontaneous vertigo

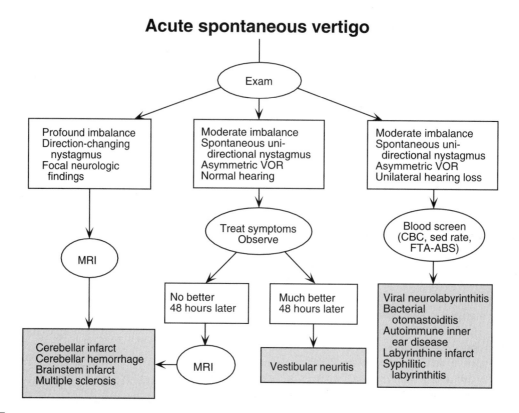

FIGURE 45 Logic for determining the cause of acute, spontaneous vertigo. TIA = transient ischemic attack; VOR = vestibulo-ocular reflex; CBC = complete blood count; sed rate = sedimentation rate; FTA-ABS = fluorescent treponemal antibody absorption test.

Patients with cerebellar infarction or hemorrhage often cannot stand or walk at all without falling.

As already noted, the history often provides information critical to deciding whether vertigo is of peripheral or central origin. The age of the patient and whether there is a history of hypertension, atherosclerosis, vascular disease, or stroke suggest whether brain infarction or hemorrhage is a consideration. Associated unilateral hearing loss or prior trauma or infection involving the ear points toward a peripheral source. On physical examination patients with peripheral vestibular lesions have impaired balance, but they are able to walk during the acute phase. By contrast, patients with central vestibular lesions often are unable to stand or take even a single step without falling. Because it is so critical, patients should try to stand and walk even though they are extremely uncomfortable and prefer to lie still in bed. Spontaneous nystagmus of peripheral origin does not change direction with gaze to either side, although it increases in amplitude with gaze in the direction of the fast phase and decreases with gaze away from the fast phase. By contrast, spontaneous nystagmus of central origin typically changes direction when the patient looks away from the direction of the fast phase. In addition, peripheral spontaneous nystagmus is inhibited with fixation, so the nystagmus usually is prominent only for the first 12 to 24 hours. Within a few days it may be inhibited completely, even with gaze in the direction of the fast phase. By contrast, spontaneous nystagmus of central origin often persists for weeks to months. Because of these features, if there is a question on presentation regarding peripheral or central origin of vertigo, the patient simply should be observed for 24 to 48 hours to see whether the course is typical of peripheral or central vestibular lesion.

Immediate magnetic resonance imaging (MRI) is indicated on a few occasions. One of these is when a patient presents with acute vertigo and profound imbalance likely caused by cerebellar infarct or hemorrhage. These central lesions must be identified as soon as possible, because both can lead to a mass effect with compression of the brain stem. If the indications are not clear after the physical examination, the patient should be observed; if the patient is no better within 24 to 48 hours, an MRI scan should be performed. Cerebellar infarction probably is the only central lesion that could masquerade as a peripheral vestibular lesion, particularly during the first few hours, during which it may be difficult to assess gait and imbalance and the spontaneous nystagmus.[21]

An MRI scan is indicated in a patient with acute-onset, prolonged vertigo who does not improve during 24 to 48 hours of observation.

Recurrent Spontaneous Attacks of Vertigo

Recurrent attacks of vertigo occur when there is a sudden temporary and largely reversible impairment of resting neural activity of one labyrinth or its central connections, with subsequent recovery to normal or near-normal function. Such attacks typically last minutes to hours rather than days and terminate not through compensation (as with prolonged attacks) but through restoration of normal neural activity. The history provides one additional key piece of information in such patients—the duration of attacks. Vertigo of vascular origin (transient ischemic attacks) typically lasts minutes, whereas peripheral inner ear causes of recurrent vertigo typically last hours. If there are focal neurologic findings on examination, one proceeds directly to an MRI (Fig. 46). It is important to keep in mind, however, that patients with vertebrobasilar transient ischemic attacks often have a completely normal neurologic examination between attacks. A screening audiogram and ENG are indicated in any patient who is having recurrent attacks of vertigo likely to be of peripheral origin (no neurologic symptoms and signs, with or without hearing loss). The diagnosis of Ménière's disease rests on finding the characteristic fluctuating low-frequency hearing loss associated with attacks of vertigo. Early in the disease process, however, hearing and vestibular function can be normal with Ménière's disease. Every patient presenting with a clinical picture typical of Ménière's disease should undergo blood screening tests to rule out the possibility of latent syphilis (congenital or acquired) and autoimmune inner ear disease.[22] Vertigo can be the only manifestation of migraine (as a migraine equivalent), but usually there is associated headache, which may or may not occur at the time of the vertigo.[23] Asymmetrical caloric responses occasionally are

Whether recurrent attacks of vertigo last for minutes or hours is an important diagnostic point.

Recurrent spontaneous attacks of vertigo

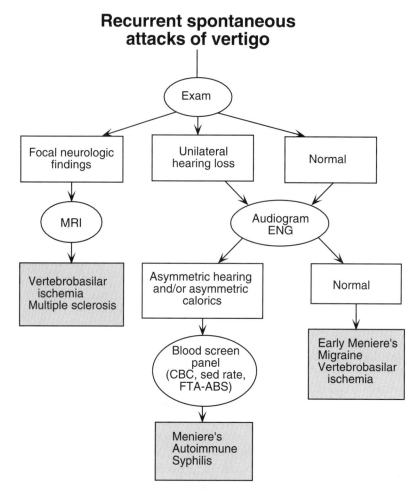

FIGURE 46 Logic for determining the cause of recurrent spontaneous attacks of vertigo. ENG = electronystagmogram; CBC = complete blood count; sed rate = sedimentation rate; FTA-ABS = fluorescent treponemal antibody absorption test.

seen with migraine, but hearing loss is infrequent. Although vertigo can be the initial symptom of multiple sclerosis, recurrent attacks of vertigo without other associated neurologic symptoms would be a rare presentation for this disorder.

Recurrent Episodes of Positional Vertigo

Positional vertigo results from a transient excitation within the vestibular pathways triggered by a position change. Since the otolith organs are the receptors sensitive to changes in the direction of gravity, positional vertigo has traditionally been attributed to lesions of the otoliths and their connections in the vestibular nuclei and cerebellum. If the semicircular canal cupula is altered in such a way that its specific gravity no longer equals that of the surrounding endolymph, however, this organ also becomes sensitive to changes in the direction of gravity and can produce positional vertigo. Structural and metabolic factors can alter the specific gravity of the cupula and produce positional vertigo. Even more important, freely moving debris within the semicircular canals can produce positional vertigo as the debris moves from one position to another under the influence of gravity.[24,25]

The history usually can separate positional vertigo from spontaneous attacks of vertigo. Patients sometimes report having vertigo for several days when what they mean is that they were susceptible to episodes of positional vertigo during that time. Positional vertigo nearly always is a benign condition that can be cured easily at the bedside, but in rare cases it can be a symptom of a central lesion, particularly one near the fourth ventricle. The diagnosis usually is clear after performing standard positional testing such as the Dix-Hallpike maneuver (see Fig. 29). If the patient exhibits the characteristic fatigable torsional positional nystagmus that lasts less than 30 seconds, the diagnosis of benign positional vertigo is made (Fig. 47). Any deviation from this characteristic nystagmus profile should raise suspicion about a central lesion. Central positional nystagmus typically is nonfatiguing and purely vertical (either upbeating or downbeating). Most cases of central positional nystagmus have other associated neurologic findings. Because there are horizontal canal variants of benign positional vertigo, transient direction-changing horizontal nystagmus induced by turning the head to the side may be of benign peripheral origin.[26] Common causes of central positional vertigo are

> *Positional testing usually can identify the cause of positional vertigo, nearly always a benign disorder.*

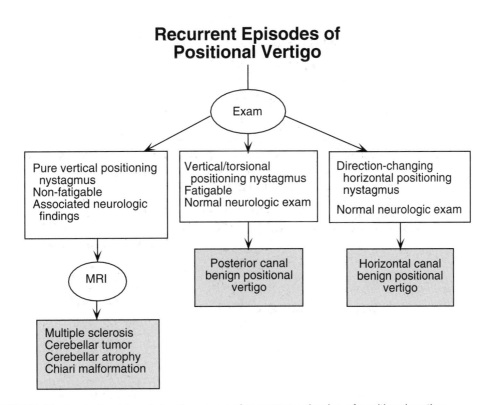

FIGURE 47   Logic for determining the cause of recurrent episodes of positional vertigo.

multiple sclerosis, cerebellar tumors, cerebellar atrophy, and Arnold-Chiari malformation.

Posttraumatic Dizziness

Dizziness is a common symptom after head trauma because both the brain and the inner ear are extremely vulnerable to blunt trauma whether or not there is an associated fracture of the skull.[27] The history is critical for determining the type of dizziness (vertigo vs. nonspecific), the duration of attacks, and the precipitating events (Fig. 48). Positional vertigo may not be seen for several days or even weeks after head trauma if the patient is severely injured and unable to move about. The **postconcussion**

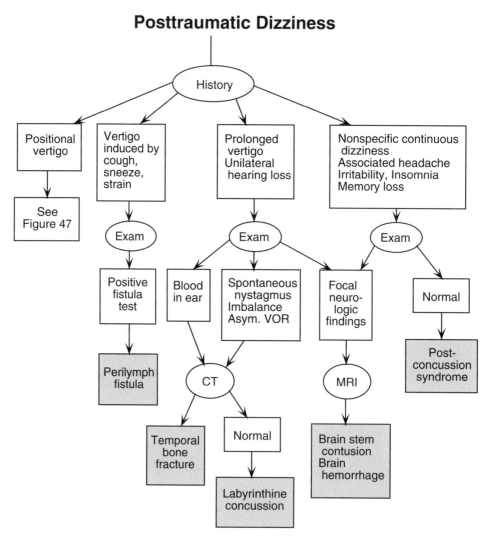

FIGURE 48 Logic for determining the cause of posttraumatic dizziness (From Baloh, RW, et al: CONTINUUM: Neurotology 2(1), p. 79. Reprinted with kind permission of the American Academy of Neurology, 1996.)

syndrome is characterized by a combination of symptoms including dizziness, headache, increased irritability, insomnia, forgetfulness, difficulty concentrating, and loss of initiative.[28,29] The dizziness is nearly always nonspecific; patients use terms such as swimming, light-headed, floating, rocking, and disoriented to describe the sensation they feel. Of course, vertigo can also be present if there is an additional labyrinthine lesion.

Persistent dizziness after blunt head trauma can pose a difficult diagnostic dilemma (Table 14). A careful neurotological examination should identify most specific syndromes that require individualized treatment. Examination of the ear may reveal evidence of a temporal bone fracture or perilymph fistula; positional testing may reveal benign positional nystagmus; neurologic examination may identify signs of brain stem damage. Quantitative auditory and vestibular function testing can be useful to document fixed deficits in the auditory and vestibular systems. Neuroimaging is usually helpful only when there are focal findings on the neurologic examination. CT scanning is most useful for evaluating the base of the skull, and MRI provides the best assessment of brain stem and cerebellar structures.

> *A careful neurotological exam is needed to identify the many causes of persistent dizziness after blunt head trauma.*

Disequilibrium without Vertigo

Patients with disequilibrium but not vertigo are a diagnostic challenge because the cause can be lesions at locations as varied as the inner ears, the peripheral nerves and muscles, and multiple sites within the CNS (Fig. 49). The act of standing and walking requires complex sensory integration and processing.[30] Vestibular, somatosensory, and visual senses all provide orienting information to the brain, and this sensory information is constantly being integrated to generate an appropriate motor response.

A careful examination should discriminate between the many

Table 14 Differential Diagnosis of Persistent Dizziness after Head Trauma

	Nature of Dizziness	Exam	Laboratory
Benign positional vertigo	Brief episodes, position induced	Fatigable positioning nystagmus	Normal
Labyrinthine concussion	Severe initially, gradual improvement	Peripheral spontaneous nystagmus	Caloric vestibular paresis, unilateral hearing loss
Perilymph fistula	Fluctuating, induced by coughing, sneezing, straining	Positive fistula test	Caloric vestibular paresis
Brain stem contusion	Severe continuous associated brain stem symptoms	Focal neurologic signs	MR scan shows focal lesions
Postconcussion syndrome	Mild continuous, associated headache, insomnia, irritability, fatigue, difficulty concentrating	Normal	Normal

Disequilibrium without vertigo

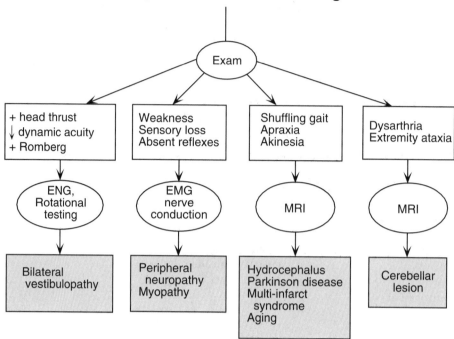

FIGURE 49 Logic for determining the cause of disequilibrium without vertigo.

causes of disequilibrium. Several bedside tests indicate bilateral vestibular loss (discussed in Chapter 5), but a definitive diagnosis requires vestibular function testing, preferably with quantitative rotational tests. Balance and gait disorders in older patients often are multifactorial. So-called **multisensory dizziness** occurs when there is a partial loss of multiple sensory inputs (e.g., diabetic peripheral neuropathy and retinopathy). The normal deterioration in gait and balance that occurs with aging can mimic potentially treatable disorders such as occult hydrocephalus, Parkinson's disease, and multi-infarct syndrome.[15] An MRI of the brain should help distinguish among these entities.

Some treatable disorders causing disequilibrium may be mistaken for the normal deterioration of aging.

References

1. Baloh RW: History. I. Patient with dizziness. In Baloh RW, and Halmagyi GM (eds): Disorders of the Vestibular System. Oxford University Press, New York, 1996.
2. Halmagyi GM: History. II. Patient with vertigo. In Baloh RW, and Halmagyi GM (eds): Disorders of the Vestibular System. Oxford University Press, New York, 1996.
3. Goodhill V: Leaking labyrinth lesions, deafness, tinnitus and dizziness. Ann Otol Rhinol Laryngol 90:99, 1981.
4. Nadol JB: Positive Hennebert's sign in Ménière's disease. Arch Otolaryngol 103:524, 1977.
5. Kaufman H: Neurally mediated syncope: Pathogenesis, diagnosis, and treatment. Neurology 45 (Suppl 5):S12, 1995.
6. Mathias CJ: Orthostatic hypotension: Causes, mechanisms, and influencing factors. Neurology 45 (Suppl 5):S5, 1995.

7. Roberston D, and Davis TL: Recent advances in the treatment of orthostatic hypotension. Neurology 45 (Suppl 5):S26, 1995.
8. Magarian GJ: Hyperventilation syndromes: Infrequently recognized common expressions of anxiety and stress. Medicine 61:219, 1982.
9. Jacob RG, Furman JM, and Balaban CD: Psychiatric aspects of vestibular disorders. In Baloh RW, and Halmagyi GM (eds): Disorders of the Vestibular System. Oxford University Press, New York, 1996.
10. Tucker GJ: Psychiatric disorders in medical practice. In Wyngarden JB, and Smith LH (eds): Cecil Textbook of Medicine, ed 18. Harcourt Brace Jovanovich, Philadelphia, 1988.
11. Katon W: Panic disorder: Epidemiology, diagnosis and treatment in primary care. J Clin Psychiatry (Suppl) 47:21, 1986.
12. Johnson MR, Lydiard RB, and Ballenger JC: Panic disorder: Pathophysiology and drug treatment. Drugs 49:328, 1995.
13. Brandt T, Huppert D, and Dieterich M: Phobic postural vertigo: A first follow-up. J Neurol 241:191, 1994.
14. Service FJ: Hypoglycemia. Med Clin North Am 79:1, 1995.
15. Baloh RW: Disequilibrium and gait disorders in older people. Rev Clin Gerontol 6:41, 1996.
16. Bloem BR, Haan J, Lagaay AM, et al.: Investigation of gait in elderly subjects over 88 years of age. J Geriatr Psychiatry Neurol 5:78, 1992.
17. Tinetti ME, Speechley M, and Ginter SF: Risk factors for falls among elderly persons living in the community. N Engl J Med 319:1701, 1988.
18. Rubenstein LZ, Robbins AS, Schulman BL, et al.: Falls and instability in the elderly. J Am Geriatr 36:266, 1988.
19. Halmagyi GM, Fattore CM, Curthoys IS, et al.: Gentamicin vestibulotoxicity. Otolaryngol Head Neck Surg 111:571, 1994.
20. Gallagher BB, Baumel IP, Mattson RH, and Woodbury SG: Primidone, diphenylhydantoin and phenobarbital: Aspects of acute and chronic toxicity. Neurology 23:145, 1973.
21. Huang CY, and Yu YL: Small cerebellar strokes may mimic labyrinthine lesions. J Neurol Neurosurg Psychiatry 48:263, 1985.
22. Andrews JC, and Honrubia V: Ménière's disease. In Baloh RW, and Halmagyi GM (eds): Disorders of the Vestibular System. Oxford University Press, New York, 1996.
23. Cutrer FM, and Baloh RW: Migraine-associated dizziness. Headache 32:300, 1992.
24. McClure JA, and Parnes LS: A cure for benign positional vertigo. In Baloh RW (ed): Bailliere's Clinical Neurology. International Practice and Research. Neurology. Bailliere Tindall, London, 1994.
25. Suzuki M, Kadir A, Hayashi N, and Takamoto M: Functional model of benign paroxysmal positional vertigo using an isolated frog semicircular canal. J Vest Res 6:121, 1996.
26. Baloh RW: Benign positional vertigo. In Baloh RW, and Halmagyi GM (eds): Disorders of the Vestibular System. Oxford University Press, New York, 1996.
27. Luxon LM: Posttraumatic vertigo. In Baloh RW, and Halmagyi GM (eds): Disorders of the Vestibular System. Oxford University Press, New York, 1996.
28. Binder LM: Persisting symptoms after mild head injury: A review of the postconcussive syndrome. J Clin Exp Neuropsychol 8:323, 1986.
29. Alexander MP: Mild traumatic brain injury: Pathophysiology, natural history, and clinical management. Neurology 45:1253, 1995.
30. Nutt JG, Marsden CD, and Thompson PD: Human walking and higher-level gait disorders, particularly in the elderly. Neurology 43:268, 1993.

9

Approach to the Patient with Tinnitus

Tinnitus is a noise in the ear that is usually audible only to the patient, although occasionally the sound can be heard by the examining physician ("objective tinnitus").[1,2] The pathophysiology of tinnitus is largely unknown. With disease of the external or the middle ear, tinnitus may result from a reduction of ambient noise, thereby allowing internal auditory signals to become more apparent. Ototoxic drugs and noise exposure presumably damage cochlear hair cells, leading to abnormal firing of primary afferents and tinnitus.[3] Central auditory mechanisms also play a role in the pathophysiology of tinnitus; often tinnitus will persist after the inner ear or cranial nerve VIII is removed, and many centrally active drugs can induce tinnitus, as discussed later.

KEY FEATURES IN THE HISTORY

Tinnitus is a symptom that can be associated with a variety of neurotological disorders that may affect the ear or the brain.[4,5] As with dizziness, the initial task of the examining physician is to obtain a detailed description of the nature of the tinnitus (Table 15). Possibly the most important single piece of information is whether the tinnitus is localized to one ear or both ears or is non-localizable. As a general rule, tinnitus that is localized to one ear

In taking the history of a patient with tinnitus, find out whether the tinnitus is localized, episodic, or rhythmic; what it sounds like; and whether there are any associated symptoms.

Table 15   **Key Features That Should Be Elicited in the History of a Patient Complaining of Tinnitus**

Location	One ear
	Both ears
	"In head"
Duration	Episodic (how long?)
	Continuous
Pitch	High (ringing, steam, wind, clicking)
	Low (roar, seashell, grinding)
Pattern	Pulsatile (synchronous with pulse)
	Blowing (synchronous with respiration)
	Circadian (increases at certain time of day)
	Steady

will have an identifiable cause, whereas tinnitus that is in both ears or is nonlocalizable often will not. If the tinnitus occurs in episodes, find out the duration and whether there are associated symptoms. The patient should try to compare the tinnitus sound to some identifiable sound in the environment. For example, typical tinnitus associated with Ménière's disease is described as a roaring sound, like listening to a seashell; the tinnitus associated with an acoustic neuroma is typically a high-pitched ringing or like the sound of steam blowing from a teakettle. If the tinnitus is rhythmic, the patient should be asked whether it is synchronous with the pulse or with respiration. Most patients with tinnitus are bothered most at night, when it is quiet and there is less background noise to mask the tinnitus. Occasionally patients will notice that their tinnitus is loudest when they are under stress or in certain situations that have been stressful in the past. Other features that are noteworthy in the history include the patient's age, the time of onset of tinnitus, associated otological complaints such as hearing loss or vertigo, associated neurologic complaints, and medication use.

The distress suffered by patients with tinnitus appears to depend on many factors, such as their predisposition to depression and the presence of other medical problems.[6] As many as 50% of patients with tinnitus suffer from depression, which is severe in approximately 10% of patients with tinnitus.[7] In some patients, tinnitus is thought to lead to depression, but in others it is thought to be a component of the patient's depression. Tinnitus can also lead to anxiety and insomnia. Each of these conditions can be treated separately even if the patient's underlying tinnitus cannot be cured (see Chapter 12).

CAUSES OF TINNITUS

The flowchart in Figure 50 summarizes the logic for distinguishing among different causes of tinnitus.

Tinnitus

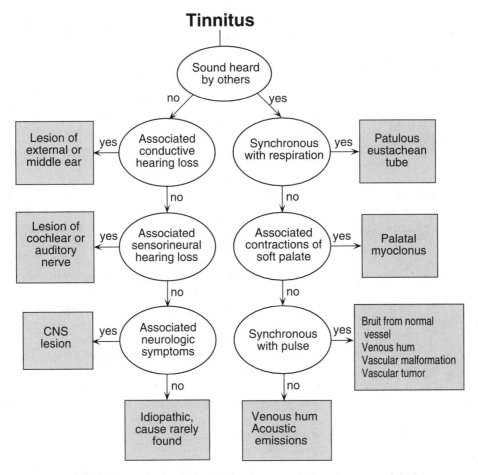

FIGURE 50   Logic for distinguishing between different causes of tinnitus.

Objective Tinnitus

Objective tinnitus can be heard when the examining physician places a stethoscope into the patient's external auditory canal. A blowing sound that coincides with inspiration, expiration, or both can result from an abnormally patent eustachian tube. This type of tinnitus is particularly common after recent weight loss or a debilitating illness. Tinnitus characterized by a series of sharp clicks heard for several seconds or minutes at a time can result from tetanic contractions of the muscles of the soft palate. These contractions can be observed by the examiner when the tinnitus is audible. Tinnitus that is pulsatory and synchronous with the heartbeat suggests the possibility of a vascular abnormality within the head or neck.[8] Aneurysms, arteriovenous malforma-tions, and vascular tumors can produce this type of tinnitus. More commonly, it results from flow in normal arteries running near the inner ear. A **venous hum** can be either a continuous machine-like sound or a "whoosh" in synchrony with the pulse.[9,10] It oc-curs when turbulent flow in the jugular bulb produces a sound

Some tinnitus that can be heard by the physician is caused by blood flow in normal arteries.

that is transmitted to the ear. Objective tinnitus can also be a sign of increased intracranial pressure, presumably because of turbulent flow in compressed veins at the base of the brain.[11] Such tinnitus is usually overshadowed by other neurologic findings. Oscillatory vibrations within the cochlea can be heard in many normal ears when one uses a special ear canal recording technique. These so-called **acoustic emissions** are audible to some subjects and may be one source of mild tonal tinnitus, particularly in a quiet environment.[12]

Subjective Tinnitus

Subjective tinnitus (heard only by the patient) can result from lesions involving the external ear canal, tympanic membrane, ossicles, cochlea, auditory nerve, brain stem, and cortex.[1,13] The description of the noise can vary from an ill-defined buzzing, ringing, hissing, or whistling to a more recognizable sound such as a cricket, seashell, or motor. The patient's description of the loudness, pitch, and duration of tinnitus can be diagnostically useful (see Table 15). The characteristic low-pitched tinnitus associated with Ménière's disease often becomes very loud immediately preceding an acute attack of vertigo and then may transiently disappear after the attack. Tinnitus with otosclerosis is also usually low pitched, described as a buzzing or roaring sound. It is usually continuous but can occasionally be intermittent or even pulsatile. In some patients with otosclerosis, the tinnitus is more disturbing than is the hearing loss. Most people experience a high-pitched ringing tinnitus after a slap across the head or close exposure to a sudden very loud noise, such as an explosion or the firing of a gun. This tinnitus usually subsides within a few hours, although occasionally, if permanent hearing loss has occurred from damage to the inner ear, a high-pitched ringing tinnitus may persist for years. Continuous bilateral high-pitched tinnitus often accompanies chronic noise-induced hearing loss, presbycusis, and hearing loss due to ototoxic drugs. Continuous unilateral high-pitched tinnitus may be the first symptom of an acoustic neuroma, preceding loss of hearing by several years.

Associated symptoms and signs are important in identifying the cause of tinnitus.

As with vertigo, the character of the tinnitus alone does not determine the site of the disturbance. For this, one must rely on associated symptoms and signs. When tinnitus results from a lesion of the external or the middle ear, it is usually accompanied by a conductive hearing loss. Patients may complain that their voice sounds hollow and other sounds are muffled. Since the masking effect of ambient noise is lost, these patients may be disturbed by normal muscular sounds such as chewing, tight closure of the eyes, or clenching of the jaws. Tinnitus caused by lesions of the cochlea or auditory nerve is usually associated with sensorineural hearing loss, with or without distortion of sounds or diplacusis. The pitch of the tinnitus often corresponds to the frequency at which the hearing loss is greatest. Tinnitus resulting from lesions within the central nervous system is usually not associated with hearing loss but is nearly always associated with other neurologic symptoms and signs.

Drug-Induced Tinnitus

As many as 50% of patients with tinnitus do not have associated hearing loss. In such patients, the cause of tinnitus can be difficult to identify. Numerous drugs can produce tinnitus without associated hearing loss (Table 16).[3,14] The anatomical site of action of these drugs in producing tinnitus is unknown, although both peripheral and central effects probably occur. Many are known to affect biogenic amine neurotransmission within the central nervous system. Such drugs might produce tinnitus by facilitating or altering the balance of transmitted signals through the central auditory pathways. When cats are given sodium salicylate to produce blood concentrations commonly associated with tinnitus in normal human subjects (0.3 to 0.6 mg/mL), the threshold of all primary afferent fibers is increased irrespective of their characteristic frequency and spontaneous activity.[15] Associated with the increase in threshold is a reduction in the tuning and dynamic range of cochlear afferent fibers typical of the response to many other ototoxic drugs. With salicylates, however, an increase in the spontaneous discharge rate occurs in those fibers whose spontaneous activity is greater than 20 spikes per second. This finding is an important exception to the general rule that damage to the cochlea depresses cochlear afferent nerve spontaneous activity.

The diagnosis of drug-induced tinnitus is usually straightforward, especially if the discontinuation of a particular medication leads to a reduction or complete resolution of the tinnitus. Generally, the development of tinnitus depends on the blood levels of the medication used and thus upon the dosage, but individuals vary widely in their susceptibility to drug-induced tinnitus. Renal function may influence tinnitus by affecting drug levels of some agents such as aminoglycosides and cisplatin. Susceptibility also depends in an unpredictable way upon any pre-existing hearing loss or simultaneous noise exposure. Patients receiving two drugs that cause tinnitus may experience a synergistic effect.

The pathophysiology of drug-induced tinnitus varies according to the agent.[3,14] Aminoglycosides irreversibly affect outer hair

Tinnitus without hearing loss may be drug-induced.

Table 16   **Commonly Used Drugs That Can Produce Tinnitus**

Caffeine
Salicylates
Quinidine
Indomethacin
Propranolol
Levodopa
Carbamazepine
Aminophylline

cells and with repeated exposure can affect inner hair cells as well. Cisplatin also irreversibly affects the outer hair cells but may also directly affect the spiral ganglion or cochlear nerve. Quinine is thought to cause irreversible damage to the organ of Corti and stria vascularis; loop diuretics also damage the stria vascularis. Salicylates cause reversible tinnitus; they are thought to impair enzymatic actions within hair cells and neurons.

WORKUP OF COMMON PRESENTATIONS OF TINNITUS

Unilateral Pulsatile Tinnitus

Unilateral pulsatile tinnitus is by far the most common type of objective tinnitus. Very often it is a benign symptom associated with normal vascular sounds. It can be the first symptom of a more serious problem, such as an arteriovenous malformation, vascular tumor, or aneurysm, however, and these processes must be ruled out before the patient can be reassured (Fig. 51). The history supplies important data regarding risk factors for vascular

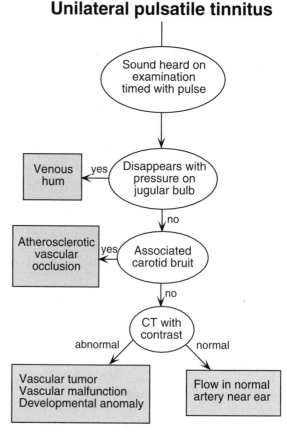

Unilateral pulsatile tinnitus

FIGURE 51   Logic for determining the cause of unilateral pulsatile tinnitus.

disease, prior transient ischemic attacks or stroke, or evidence of occlusive vascular disease in other parts of the body. Pulsatile tinnitus developing after head trauma suggests the possibility of an arteriovenous malformation, particularly involving the cavernous sinus.[16] A venous hum can be a continuous, machinelike sound, a pulsatile sound, or some combination of these two sounds. It can be eliminated temporarily by gentle pressure on the neck that occludes the jugular vein but not the arterial blood flow. Atherosclerotic vascular disease can cause a carotid bruit that is transmitted to the nearby inner ear.[17]

Pulsatile tinnitus beginning after head trauma may indicate an arteriovenous malformation.

The evaluation of a patient with pulsatile tinnitus often includes a CT scan with contrast. This study can show bony erosion and will provide information about the vascularity of any structure identified. MRI and MR angiography may provide additional information regarding the features of an identified lesion. Traditional angiography is still the gold standard for documenting vascular tumors and vascular malformations that cause pulsatile tinnitus.

Chronic Unilateral Subjective Tinnitus

When a patient presents with unilateral subjective tinnitus, the relevant history will include the patient's age, type of onset, duration of symptoms, and presence or absence of associated auditory, vestibular, or neurologic symptoms (Fig. 52). Tinnitus associated with sudden deafness is usually due to labyrinthitis or labyrinthine concussion. A history of trauma, infection, or systemic illness may be critical. The external auditory canals should be examined carefully to rule out impacted cerumen, infection, or obvious results of trauma. The key laboratory test in every patient complaining of unilateral tinnitus is the audiogram, because the pattern of hearing loss (when present) provides important diagnostic information (see Fig. 39).

Patients with subjective tinnitus should have an audiogram to determine the pattern of their hearing loss, if any.

Any patient in whom there is a documented progressive unilateral sensorineural hearing loss should have an MRI with contrast to rule out an acoustic neuroma or other tumor involving the acoustic nerve (see Fig. 73). Although more than 95% of patients with acoustic neuroma present with unilateral hearing loss, patients occasionally present with unilateral tinnitus without hearing loss.[18] In that case, an abnormal brain stem auditory evoked response indicates involvement of the acoustic nerve and leads to an MRI with contrast. Because acoustic neuromas invariably are slow growing and rarely present with normal hearing, it is reasonable to simply follow patients who present with unilateral tinnitus and normal hearing by repeating audiograms every 3 to 6 months. If evidence of a progressive hearing loss develops, then an MRI with contrast is indicated.

Causes of periodic unilateral tinnitus such as Ménière's disease, autoimmune disease, and perilymph fistula are usually readily evident based on the combination of symptoms and signs (see Chapter 10).

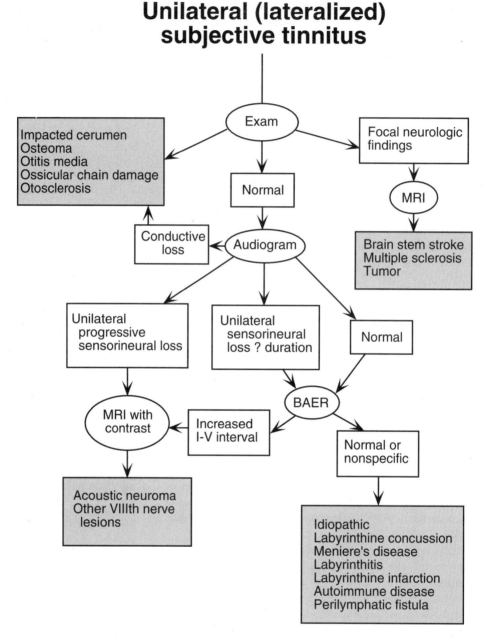

Unilateral (lateralized) subjective tinnitus

■ **FIGURE 52** Logic for determining the cause of unilateral subjective tinnitus.

Chronic Bilateral Subjective Tinnitus

Patients with bilateral subjective tinnitus and hearing loss related to noise exposure or presbycusis may get relief from amplification.

Unlike unilateral subjective tinnitus, bilateral tinnitus rarely has a treatable cause (Fig. 53). One exception would be tinnitus caused by a drug, which could be identified and discontinued (see Table 16). The key laboratory test in assessing patients with bilateral tinnitus (as for unilateral) is the audiogram. By far the most common abnormalities identified are a bilateral notched (at 4000 Hz) sensorineural hearing loss caused by noise exposure[19] or a bilat-

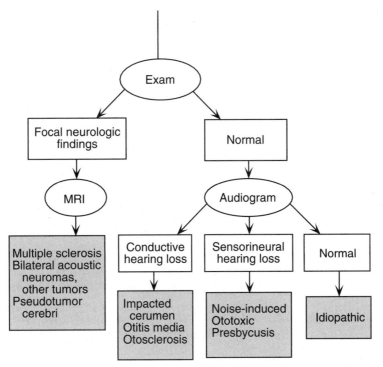

■ **FIGURE 53**   Logic for determining the cause of bilateral subjective tinnitus.

eral symmetrical, sloping sensorineural hearing loss typical of presbycusis. Patients with both of these disorders often complain of bilateral tinnitus. Sometimes amplification improves not only hearing but also tinnitus, probably because it introduces background sounds that help mask the tinnitus.[17] Neurologic causes of bilateral tinnitus are rare.

In many patients, the cause of tinnitus is never found despite a thorough evaluation. Tinnitus in such patients is nonlocalized, nonpulsatile, and continuous. Some patients with idiopathic tinnitus tolerate their symptoms adequately and continue to cope with their activities of daily living without interruption. Many such patients, however, are greatly distressed by their symptoms and may focus upon their tinnitus, with adverse effects on their work and family lives. Such patients rate their tinnitus as louder even though objective measures of tinnitus loudness using masking do not reveal that their tinnitus is louder than that of other, less distressed patients.[20]

References

1. Hazell JWP (ed): Tinnitus. Churchill Livingstone, Edinburgh, 1987.
2. Douek E: Classification of tinnitus. In CIBA Foundation Symposium No. 85, London, 1981.

3. Brown D, Penny JE, Henley CH, et al.: Ototoxic drugs and noise. In CIBA Foundation Symposium No. 85, London, 1981.

4. Vernon J: Assessment of the tinnitus patient. In Hazell JWP (ed): Tinnitus. Churchill Livingstone, Edinburgh, 1987.

5. Lechtenberg R, and Shulman A: The neurologic implications of tinnitus. Arch Neurol 41:717, 1984.

6. Meikle MB, Vernon J, and Johnson RM: The perceived severity of tinnitus: Some observations concerning a large population of tinnitus clinic patients. Otolaryngol Head Neck Surg 92:689, 1984.

7. McKenna L, Hallam RS, and Hinchcliffe R: The prevalence of psychological disturbance in neuro-otology outpatients. Clin Otolaryngol 16:452, 1991.

8. Sismanis A, and Smoker WR: Pulsatile tinnitus: Recent advances in diagnosis. Laryngoscope 104:681, 1994.

9. Ward PH, Babin R, Calcaterra TC, and Konrad HR: Operative treatment of surgical lesions with objective tinnitus. Ann Otol Rhinol Laryngol 84:473, 1975.

10. Golueke PJ, Panetta T, Scalfani S, and Verghese G: Tinnitus originating from an abnormal jugular bulb: Treatment by jugular vein ligation. J Vasc Surg 6:248, 1987.

11. Murphy TP: Otologic manifestations of pseudotumor cerebri. J Otolaryngol 20:258, 1991.

12. Penner MJ: Linking spontaneous otoacoustic emissions and tinnitus. Br J Audiol 26:115, 1992.

13. Jackson PD: Tinnitus. In Bagley HA (ed): Audiology and Audiologic Medicine. Oxford University Press, Oxford, 1981.

14. McFadden D: Tinnitus: Facts, theories and treatments. National Academic Press, Washington, DC, 1982.

15. Evans EF, Wilson JP, and Borerwe TA: Animal models of tinnitus. In CIBA Foundation Symposium No. 85, London, 1981.

16. Vernon JA, and Press LS: Characteristics of tinnitus induced by head injury. Arch Otolaryngol Head Neck Surg 120:547, 1994.

17. Louwrens HD, Botha J, and Van der Merwe DM: Subjective pulsatile tinnitus cured by carotid endarterectomy. S Afr Med J 75:496, 1989.

18. Jackler RK: Acoustic neuroma (vestibular schwannoma). In Jackler RE, and Brackmann DE (eds): Neurotology. C.V. Mosby, St. Louis, 1994.

19. Phoon WH, Lee HS, and Chia SE: Tinnitus in noise-exposed workers. Occup Med 43:35, 1993.

20. Schleuning AJ, Johnson RM, and Vernon JA: Evaluation of a tinnitus masking program: A follow-up study of 589 patients. Ear Hear 1:71, 1980.

Part III

Diagnosis and Treatment

10

Common Neurotological Disorders

Chapter Outline

INFECTIONS OF THE EAR AND THE TEMPORAL BONE

Infections of the ear and the temporal bone are a common cause of dizziness and hearing loss, particularly in children. Either infected (**suppurative otitis**) or noninfected (**serous otitis**) fluid accumulates in the middle ear, impairing conduction of airborne sound. Since the air cavity of the middle ear is in direct connection with the mastoid air cells, infection can spread throughout the pneumatized parts of the temporal bone (see Fig. 1). Figure 54 summarizes typical patterns of progression of middle ear infections.

Acute Otitis Media

Symptoms	Rapid onset of ear pain and pressure, hearing loss
Signs	Inflamed tympanic membrane, fluid or pus in middle ear, or both
Laboratory	Positive cultures (spontaneous otorrhea, myringotomy, or nasopharynx) *Audiometry:* Conductive hearing loss, flat tympanogram
Management	Initial empiric antibiotic therapy: Amoxicillin; revised antibiotic therapy based on culture and sensitivity tests

Persistent acute otitis media can lead to acute otomastoiditis.

Inflammation of the middle ear probably accompanies every viral upper respiratory tract infection (URI). The nasal, paranasal, and pharyngeal mucositis spreads to involve the eustachian tubes and middle ear mucosa, producing a **tubotympanitis**.[1] As noted in Chapter 1, the mucosa of the pharyngeal end of the eustachian tube is continuous with the mucociliary system of the middle ear. Tubotympanitis accompanying most URIs is transitory and subsides without significant sequelae. In a few cases, however, a secondary bacterial superinfection produces acute bacterial otitis media.[2,3] Common etiologic organisms are *Haemophilus influenzae* in infants and young children and *Streptococcus pneumoniae* in older children and adults.[4] Acute otitis media commonly progresses to spontaneous tympanic membrane rupture and otorrhea. Persistent acute otitis media can lead to secretory otitis media or to

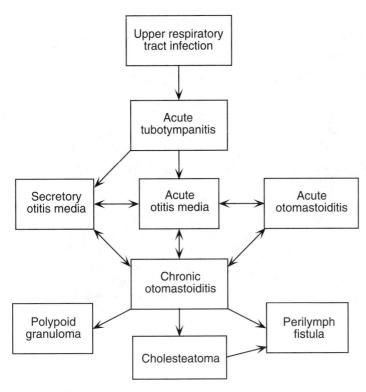

FIGURE 54   Typical patterns of progression of middle ear infections.

acute otomastoiditis. The most direct route for infection to spread into the mastoid is through the aditus ad antrum (see Fig. 1).

Chronic Otomastoiditis

Symptoms	Chronic otorrhea, ear pain, and hearing loss
Signs	Pus in external canal, perforation of tympanic membrane (particularly in pars flaccida region) (see Figs. 2 and 3), annular bone erosion, cholesteatoma, or granuloma may be visible in the epitympanic region of the middle ear
Laboratory	*Audiometry:* Conductive hearing loss, restricted or flat tympanogram, absent stapedius reflex *CT:* Nonpneumatized or poorly pneumatized mastoid, haziness of air spaces, bony erosion from cholesteatoma (Fig. 55) Positive cultures of chronic otorrhea
Management	Combined medical-surgical; antibiotics based on culture and sensitivity tests; surgical removal of granuloma or cholesteatoma combined with mastoidectomy, tympanoplasty, and ossiculoplasty as necessary

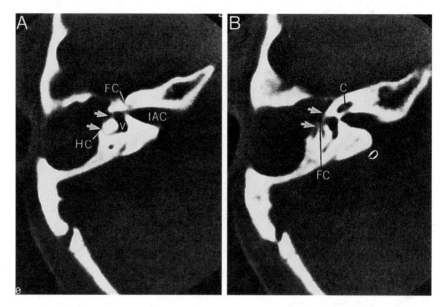

FIGURE 55   CT scan of the temporal bone in a patient with a cholesteatoma eroding the wall of the horizontal semicircular canal (*A*) and the facial canal (*B*). Arrows point toward area of bony erosion. FC = facial canal; HC = horizontal semicircular canal; V = vestibule; IAC = internal auditory canal. (Courtesy William Hanafee, M.D., and Sven Larsen, M.D., Radiology, UCLA).

Bony erosion from a cholesteatoma may produce conductive hearing loss and episodic vertigo.

Chronic otomastoiditis results from untreated or nonresponsive acute otomastoiditis or secretory otitis media.[5] In addition to the conductive hearing loss common with acute infection, ears with chronic infection have an increased incidence of sensorineural hearing loss.[6] The pathology of chronic otomastoiditis is characterized by thickened edematous mucosa, with obliteration of the mastoid air cell lumens, perivascular fibrosis, and osteitis.[7] Polypoid **granulomas** composed of hyperplastic mucosa may fill the mastoid antrum, extend into the middle ear, and extrude through a tympanic membrane perforation into the external auditory canal. Keratinizing squamous epithelium (**cholesteatoma**) can invade the middle ear and other pneumatized areas of the temporal bone through a chronic perforation in the tympanic membrane.[8] Cholesteatomas usually develop in the epitympanic space after penetrating a perforation in the pars flaccida region of the tympanic membrane (see Fig. 3B). From here they extend posteriorly into the antrum, into the central mastoid tract, or inferiorly into the middle ear to erode the ossicles and bony labyrinth, producing a mixed conductive hearing loss and vertigo (see Fig. 55). A cholesteatoma may accumulate slowly for years or may develop rapidly with a recurrent infection. When infected, the cholesteatoma may erode through the temporal bone into the intracranial cavity, producing central nervous system (CNS) symptoms and signs. Also with chronic otomastoiditis, a fistula may develop in the bony labyrinth, producing an artificial communication between the perilymph and the middle ear. The fistula is caused by either progressive rarefying osteitis or erosion by a cholesteatoma (see Fig. 55). Patients with a perilymph fistula experience incapacitating episodes of vertigo when they sneeze or cough because the sudden change in middle ear pressure is transmitted directly to the inner ear (see Perilymph Fistula, p. 180).

Malignant External Otitis

Symptoms   Subacute onset of otorrhea, hearing loss, pain, facial weakness

Signs   Pus in external canal, ipsilateral hearing loss, facial paralysis

Laboratory   Evidence of systemic illness (usually diabetes mellitus)
                Audiometry: Conductive or combined conductive-sensorineural hearing loss
                CT: Increased air cell density and trabecular erosion of mastoid
                Cultures positive for *Pseudomonas*

Management   Combined medical-surgical (Fig. 56)[9,10]

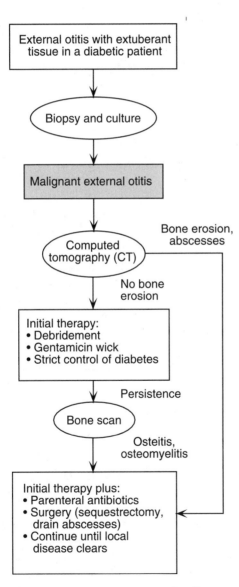

FIGURE 56   Algorithm for the management of malignant external otitis. (Adapted from Smith, PG and Lucente, FE: External ear infections. In Cummings CW, et al (eds): *Otolaryngology—Head and Neck Surgery,* ed 2. C.V. Mosby, St. Louis, 1986, with permission.)

Elderly diabetic patients are susceptible to malignant external otitis.

Otitis externa, usually a benign disorder, produces in elderly diabetic patients a debilitating disease called **malignant external otitis**.[10,11] It typically begins with a nonspecific infection of the external ear canal, resulting in complaints of pain, drainage, and fullness of the ear. The pain becomes severe and continuous as the infection spreads to contiguous soft tissues and adjacent bony structures. The invading organism is nearly always *Pseudomonas aeruginosa*. The organism invades the junction of the cartilaginous and osseous portions of the external auditory canal and spreads to the temporo-occipital bones. The most common neurologic sequela is involvement of the facial nerve in the fallopian canal or at the stylomastoid foramen. Occasionally multiple cranial nerves are compressed extradurally, and in rare cases the infection spreads across the dura to produce a purulent meningitis.

Intracranial Complications of Otitic Infection

Symptoms   Fever, ear pain, and headache persist despite adequate antibiotic treatment of otitic infection

Signs   May be minimal; meningismus, focal or generalized seizures, focal neurologic deficits

Laboratory   *Lumbar puncture:* Increased protein and cells, positive culture
CT: Bone erosion, collections of pus within the intracranial cavity, thrombosis of the venous sinuses
MRI: Small collections of extradural pus and early stages of brain abscess formation that can be missed with CT

Management   Eradicate infection with appropriate antibiotics, establish adequate drainage, excise infected tissue[12]

Infants age 2 years or younger with acute otitis media are the most frequent victims of meningitis resulting from the intracranial extension of infection from the temporal bone.

Extension of infection from the temporal bone into the cranial cavity demands rapid diagnosis and effective therapy to prevent permanent neurologic sequelae or death (Fig. 57). Complications can result directly either from acute otitis media and mastoiditis or from chronic otomastoiditis and bone destruction. Although the incidence of morbidity and mortality with CNS complications of ear infections has markedly decreased in the antibiotic era, these disorders have not disappeared. Of the complications, meningitis is most common, usually resulting from acute otitis media in infants 2 years of age or younger (Table 17).[13]

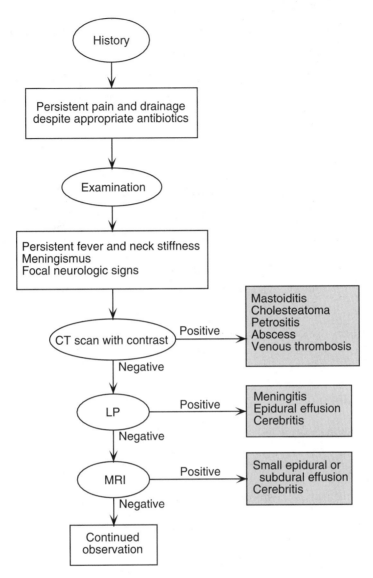

FIGURE 57 Logic for deciding the cause of intracranial complications of ear infections. CT = computerized tomography, MRI = magnetic resonance imaging; LP = lumbar puncture. (Adapted from Baloh, RW and Honrubia, V: *Clinical Neurophysiology of the Vestibular System,* ed 2. F.A. Davis, Philadelphia, 1990, p. 198.)

Table 17 **CNS Complications of 100 Ear Infections in One Hospital over a 20-Year Period**

Meningitis	76
Brain abscess	6
Subdural effusion	5
Lateral sinus thrombosis	5
Otitic hydrocephalus	5
Subdural empyema	3
	100

Adapted from Gower and McGuirt.[13]

Infection within the temporal bone can reach the intracranial space via three routes: direct extension, hematogenous spread, and thrombophlebitis. Extracranial subperiosteal abscesses, intracranial extradural abscesses, and sigmoid sinus thrombophlebitis almost always result from a direct extension of the temporal bone infection.[14] Subdural and brain abscesses may also result from direct extension along the soft tissue planes through the petromastoid canal to the posterior fossa or along the petrosquamous suture line to the middle fossa. In and around the temporal bone is a rich network of veins that directly communicates with extracranial, intracranial, and cranial diploic veins. Thrombophlebitis of any of these veins may spread to the others, causing osteomyelitis of the calvaria or brain abscesses at some distance from the temporal bone. Meningitis, particularly in young children, typically results from hematogenous dissemination. The frequent association of acute otitis media, pneumonia, and meningitis is probably due to the fact that all three diseases are caused by a systemic bacterial infection that has entered via the upper respiratory tract.

Chronic bacterial otomastoiditis produces meningitis by direct extension through bone and dura or through the inner ear via a labyrinthine fistula produced by a cholesteatoma.

Toxic (Serous) Labyrinthitis

Symptoms	Subtle hearing loss, rarely vertigo and imbalance
Signs	Unilateral hearing loss, acute otitis media
Laboratory	*Audiometry:* High-frequency sensorineural hearing loss
	ENG: May show decreased caloric response
	Positive culture of pus from middle ear
Management	Antibiotics based on culture and sensitivity tests

Serous labyrinthitis is a common complication of acute or chronic middle ear infections.

Serous labyrinthitis is probably the single most common complication of acute or chronic middle ear infections.[12] With acute otitis media, small molecules such as bacterial toxins and enzymes rapidly diffuse through the round window into the scala tympani. Acute and chronic inflammatory cells also infiltrate the round window, and a fine serofibrinous precipitate forms just medial to the round window membrane. The toxins, inflammatory cells, or both may penetrate the basilar membrane and invade the endolymph at the basal turn of the cochlea. Such changes probably explain the high incidence of high-frequency sensorineural hearing loss in patients with chronic otitis media.[15] A more rapid onset of serous labyrinthitis causes complete sensorineural hearing loss along with vestibular symptoms including episodic vertigo and unsteadiness. Ménière's disease can be a sequela of both serous and suppurative labyrinthitis.[16]

Bacterial (Suppurative) Labyrinthitis

Symptoms   Acute-onset deafness, vertigo, nausea, and vomiting

Signs   Unilateral or bilateral absent hearing, spontaneous nystagmus, unsteady gait

Laboratory   *Audiometry:* Profound unilateral (occasionally bilateral) sensorineural hearing
                        loss
                        ENG: Spontaneous nystagmus most prominent with eyes closed or opened in
                        darkness, absent response to caloric stimulation on side of hearing loss
                        Positive cultures: Either pus from middle ear (acute otitis media) or infected CSF
                        (meningitis)

Management   Antibiotics based on culture and sensitivity tests
                        Symptomatic treatment of vertigo (see Chapter 11)

Acute suppurative labyrinthitis has become relatively rare since the introduction of antibiotics. If it is a direct complication of middle ear disease, it is more likely to arise from a chronic otitis media and mastoiditis than from an acute middle ear infection. The most common port of entry of bacteria into the inner ear, however, is from the spinal fluid in a patient with meningitis.[12] Patients with bacterial meningitis develop labyrinthitis when bacteria enter the perilymphatic space by way of the cochlear aqueduct or internal auditory canal (Fig. 58).[16] Meningogenic bacterial labyrinthitis is usually bilateral, whereas direct invasion from a chronic otitic infection is almost always unilateral. The most common route for a direct bacterial invasion of the labyrinth is via a horizontal semicircular canal fistula from a cholesteatoma (see Fig. 55).

> *Bacterial infection of the inner ear, now relatively rare, most often follows meningitis.*

Viral Neurolabyrinthitis

Symptoms   Subacute-onset hearing loss and tinnitus and/or vertigo, nausea, and vomiting

Signs   Unilateral hearing loss, spontaneous nystagmus, unsteady gait

Laboratory   *Audiometry:* Unilateral sensorineural hearing loss
                        ENG: Spontaneous nystagmus most prominent with eyes closed or opened in
                        darkness; vestibular paresis on bithermal caloric test
                        MRI may show contrast enhancement of the eighth nerve or parts of labyrinth

Management   Consider brief course of high-dose steroids[17]; no data on antiviral agents
                        Symptomatic treatment of vertigo (see Chapter 11)

Viral neurolabyrinthitis may be part of a systemic viral illness such as measles, mumps, or infectious mononucleosis, or it may be an isolated infection of the labyrinth, eighth nerve, or both, without systemic involvement.[18] Of the thousands of infants born

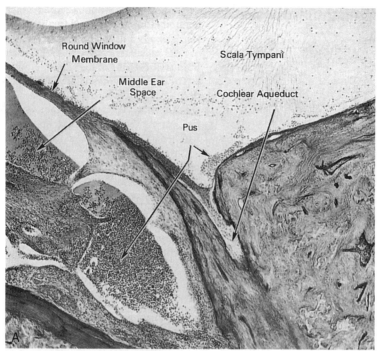

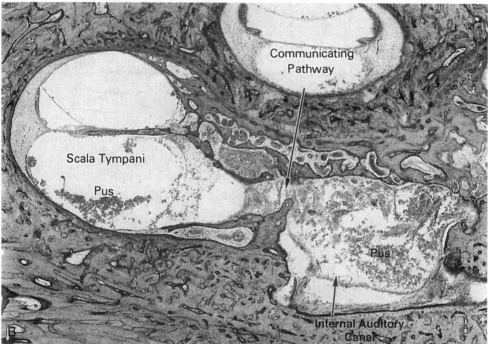

FIGURE 58   Histopathoogical sections of the temporal bone from a patient with pneumococcal otitis media, labyrinthitis, and meningitis. Polymorphonuclear leukocytes fill the cochlear aqueduct (*A*) and the internal auditory canal (*B*), the two potential communicating pathways between the inner ear and the cerebrospinal fluid. (From Schuknecht, HF: *Pathology of the Ear.* Harvard University Press, Cambridge, MA, 1974, with permission.)

deaf every year, about 20% are thought to be victims of congenital viral infections. More than 4000 persons in the United States are stricken each year with **sudden deafness**, a unilateral (infrequently bilateral) sensorineural hearing loss of subacute onset, presumed to be of viral origin in most cases.[19] A like number of individuals are stricken with the acute onset of intense vertigo (**vestibular neuronitis** or **vestibular neuritis**) unaccompanied by neurologic or audiological symptoms and also presumed to be of viral origin.[20] Despite the strong suspicion of a viral origin for these common neurotological disorders, proof of a viral pathophysiology in a given case is difficult to obtain.

A viral cause is likely for an acute-onset intense vertigo without neurologic or audiological symptoms.

Epidemiological evidence supports a viral cause in most patients with either sudden deafness or vestibular neuritis.[18] A large percentage of such patients report an upper respiratory tract illness within 1 to 2 weeks prior to the onset of symptoms. Both syndromes occur in epidemics, may affect several members of the same family, and erupt more commonly in the spring and early summer. Many different viruses have been clinically associated with cases of sudden deafness and vestibular neuritis (Table 18), but usually evidence that these viruses cause the symptoms is circumstantial.

The most convincing case for a viral cause of these isolated auditory and vestibular syndromes comes from pathological studies showing isolated viral involvement of the cochlea and auditory nerve in patients with sudden deafness and of the vestibular end organs and vestibular nerve in patients with vestibular neuritis (Fig. 59).[17,18,21] The atrophy of the nerves and end organs is identical to that associated with well-documented viral disorders (such as mumps or measles). These pathological studies are supported by experimental studies in animals, where it has been shown that several viruses will selectively infect the labyrinth or eighth nerve.[22]

The diagnosis of viral neurolabyrinthitis rests on finding the characteristic clinical profile along with laboratory evidence of peripheral auditory or vestibular dysfunction in the absence of neurologic symptoms and signs. When the hearing loss is partial, it tends to be most prominent in the high frequencies, consistent with neuropathological studies demonstrating the greatest degree of damage in the basilar turn of the cochlea.[23] Patients with vestibular neuritis often have hearing loss in the ultrahigh-

Table 18   Viruses That Have Been Clinically Associated with Hearing Loss, Vertigo, or Both

Cytomegalovirus	Hepatitis
Rubella	Adenovirus
Mumps	Influenza
Rubeola	Parainfluenza
Varicella-zoster	Poliomyelitis
Herpes simplex	Coxsackievirus
Epstein-Barr	Lymphocytic choriomeningitis
Variola	Yellow fever

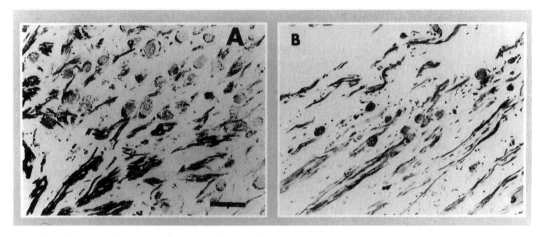

FIGURE 59 Pathological changes associated with vestibular neuritis. Histological sections through Scarpa's ganglia (*A* = normal side; *B* = abnormal side) from a patient with a typical episode of vestibular neuritis 9 years earlier. There is a marked loss of neurons and myelinated fibers in *B*. Remaining neurons are shrunken and darkly staining. Toluidine blue, bar = 100 μm (From Baloh, RW, et al.: Vestibular neuritis: Clinical-pathological correlation. Otolaryngol Head Neck Surg 114:586, 1996, with permission.)

frequency range, suggesting that the auditory end organ may be involved to a minor degree even though clinically silent.[24] Similarly, vestibular abnormalities have been identified on electronystagmography (ENG) in patients with sudden deafness but without associated vestibular symptoms.[25]

Herpes Zoster Oticus (Ramsay Hunt Syndrome)

Symptoms   Subacute onset of deep burning pain in ear, facial weakness, vertigo, hearing loss

Signs   Vesicles in external auditory canal (Fig. 60), unilateral facial paralysis,
                spontaneous nystagmus (disappears in a few days), unilateral hearing loss

Laboratory   Culture herpes zoster from vesicle fluid
                Audiometry: Sensorineural hearing loss, abnormal BAER or stapedius reflex,
                or both
                ENG: Spontaneous nystagmus most prominent with eyes closed or opened in
                darkness; vestibular paresis on bithermal caloric test

Management   Acyclovir, 1 g/day × 10 days[26]
                Symptomatic treatment of vertigo (see Chapter 11)
                Facial nerve reconstruction surgery or crossover anastomosis to spinal accessory
                nerve, hypoglossal nerve, or branches of the facial nerve on the opposite side
                if function does not return

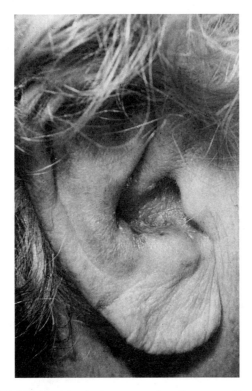

FIGURE 60   Vesicles in the external auditory canal in a patient with herpes zoster oticus.

A good example of a viral syndrome involving the eighth nerve is herpes zoster oticus. Presumably the zoster virus remains dormant in the ganglia associated with the seventh and eighth nerves and is reactivated during a period of lowered immunity. Most patients have a history of chicken pox in childhood. The patient initially develops a deep, burning pain in the ear, followed a few days later by vesicular eruption in the external auditory canal and concha (see Fig. 60).[27] Some time after the onset of pain, either before or after the vesicular eruption, the patient may develop hearing loss, vertigo, and facial weakness. These symptoms may occur singly or collectively. A few patients with idiopathic facial palsy (**Bell's palsy**) have a rise in complement fixation antibodies to zoster antigen. The pathological findings in patients with herpes zoster oticus consist of perivascular, perineural, and intraneural round-cell infiltration in the seventh nerve and both divisions of the eighth nerve.[28] Although the herpetic external otitis is self-limiting, the seventh and eighth nerve damage is often profound and irreversible.

A deep burning pain and the eruption of vesicles in the outer ear suggest herpes zoster oticus, which often irreversibly damages nerves VII and VIII.

Syphilitic Labyrinthitis

Symptoms   Hearing loss, tinnitus, and vertigo, often with associated ear pressure; begins
    unilateral, fluctuating; progresses to bilateral over months

Signs   Interstitial keratitis (Fig. 61); other manifestations of congenital syphilis
    (Hutchinson's teeth, saddle nose, frontal bossing, rhagades)
    Bilateral hearing loss, spontaneous nystagmus (transient)

Laboratory   VDRL positive (75% of cases)[29]
    FTA-ABS positive (95–100% of cases)[29]
    Audiometry: Bilateral sensorineural hearing loss, recruitment present early in
    course
    ENG: Spontaneous nystagmus with eyes closed or opened in darkness, bilateral
    decreased caloric responses
    CSF: Usually normal; may be increased protein level and pleocytosis

Management   High-dose penicillin (20 million units per day IV × 10–14 days or 2.4 million
    units weekly IM × 3 mo)[30,31]
    Steroids (prednisone, 60–100 mg per day × 10 days, then taper; maintenance dose
    if necessary)[30,31]

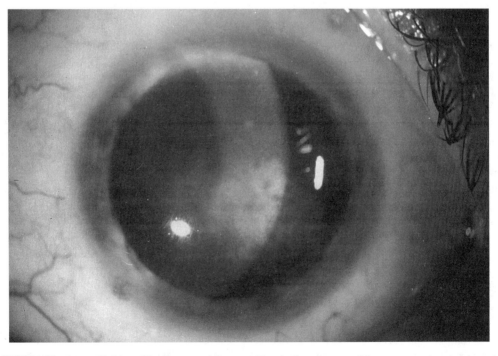

FIGURE 61   Interstitial keratitis. Dense white opacities in the stroma of the cornea stand out against the dark background of the dilated pupil. The wide beam of the slit lamp illuminates opacities in the central area of the cornea. Milder cases can be identified only with the slit lamp.

Both congenital and acquired syphilitic infections produce temporal bone osteitis and labyrinthitis as a late manifestation.[30,31] The incidence of new cases of congenital syphilis progressively declined from 1930 to 1968 but appears to have stabilized since 1968. Furthermore, after a long period of decline, new cases of acquired syphilis are again on the increase, so we might expect an increased incidence of otological manifestations in the future. The time of onset of congenital syphilitic labyrinthitis is anywhere from the first to seventh decade, with the peak incidence in the fourth and fifth decades. Acquired syphilitic labyrinthitis rarely occurs before the fourth decade and has a peak incidence in the fifth and sixth decades. The congenital variety is often associated with other stigmata of congenital syphilis. Of these, interstitial keratitis is by far the most common, occurring in about 90% of patients (see Fig. 61).[30] Pathological changes in the labyrinth are similar in the congenital and acquired varieties, consisting of inflammatory infiltration of the membranous labyrinth and osteitis of all three layers of the otic capsule.[16] A combination of hydrops of the membranous labyrinth and atrophy of the cochlear and vestibular end organs resembles the pathological findings in idiopathic Ménière's disease.

> *Interstitial keratitis can be seen in about 90% of patients with syphilitic labyrinthitis, which most commonly appears in the fourth, fifth, or sixth decades of life.*

VASCULAR DISORDERS

Vertebrobasilar insufficiency (VBI) is a common cause of vertigo in the elderly. Whether the vertigo originates from ischemia of the labyrinth, brain stem, or both structures is not always clear, because the blood supply to the labyrinth, eighth nerve, and vestibular nuclei originates from the same source, the vertebrobasilar circulation (Fig. 62). As indicated in Chapter 2, the internal auditory artery, usually a branch of the anterior inferior cerebellar artery, supplies the eighth nerve and labyrinth. The anterior inferior cerebellar artery also supplies the rostral part of the vestibular nuclei, and the posterior inferior cerebellar artery supplies the caudal part of the vestibular nuclei.

Labyrinthine Ischemia and Infarction

Symptoms	Acute vertigo, nausea and vomiting, and/or hearing loss May be preceded by TIAs within the vertebrobasilar system
Signs	Spontaneous nystagmus, imbalance, hearing loss
Laboratory	*Vascular risk factors:* Hypertension, diabetes mellitus, hypercholesterolemia, hypercoagulation *Audiometry:* Unilateral sensorineural hearing loss *ENG:* Unilateral absent caloric response
Management	Control risk factors, consider antiplatelet drugs Symptomatic treatment of vertigo, vestibular compensation exercises

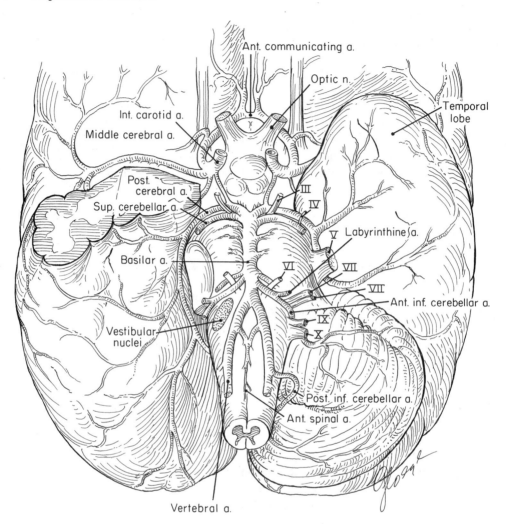

FIGURE 62 Vertebrobasilar circulation. The stippled area denotes the location of the vestibular nuclei. In addition to the brain stem, labyrinths, and cerebellum, the vertebrobasilar circulation supplies the inferomedial part of the temporal lobes (including the hippocampus) and the occipital lobes via the posterior cerebral arteries. The latter accounts for the frequent occurrence of visual symptoms with vertebrobasilar insufficiency.

Sudden-onset unilateral deafness without vertigo or brain stem signs in a patient with vascular disease may be due to ischemia.

After supplying all of the eighth nerve, the labyrinthine artery, which is about 200 μm in diameter, divides into two main branches to supply the auditory and vestibular labyrinth (see Fig. 7). Complete occlusion of the labyrinthine artery leads to a sudden, profound loss of both auditory and vestibular function. The role of vascular occlusion in the production of sudden deafness without vertigo is controversial.[32] There is little reason to suspect that unilateral deafness in a young, healthy individual is caused by vascular occlusion. Most of these cases are probably due to viral infections. The sudden onset of deafness without vertigo or brain stem signs in a patient with known vascular disease or hypercoagulation syndrome, however, should suggest the possibility of ischemia within the distribution of the common cochlear artery or one of its branches. Sudden deafness (reversible or permanent) has been reported in patients with fat emboli, thromboangiitis obliterans, and macroglobulinemia.[33] Atherosclerotic occlusive disease is also associated with sudden deafness, but pathological confirmation of the site of vascular occlusion is often lacking.

Ischemia confined to the anterior vestibular artery distribution can result in transient episodes of vertigo or prolonged vertigo due to infarction of the vestibular labyrinth. Transient episodes are often associated with hyperviscosity syndromes such as polycythemia, macroglobulinemia, and sickle cell anemia.[34] The clinical picture of vestibular labyrinth infarction is that of a sudden onset of vertigo without hearing loss or brain stem symptoms. After recovering from the acute manifestations, patients may go on to develop typical benign positional vertigo months to years later.[35] Presumably ischemic necrosis of the utricular macule leads to free-floating otoconial debris that makes its way into the posterior semicircular canal. Such patients respond to the particle repositioning maneuver, as with other causes of benign positional vertigo (see p. 166).

Labyrinthine Hemorrhage

Symptoms	Acute-onset vertigo, nausea and vomiting, and hearing loss
Signs	Spontaneous nystagmus, gait unsteadiness, and hearing loss
	Underlying bleeding diathesis, usually leukemia[36]
Laboratory	*Audiometry:* Unilateral sensorineural deafness
	ENG: Spontaneous nystagmus increases with loss of fixation, absent caloric response on side of hearing loss
Management	Symptomatic treatment of vertigo (see Chapter 11)
	Treat underlying bleeding diathesis

Spontaneous hemorrhage into the inner ear typically occurs in patients with an underlying bleeding diathesis. Such patients experience the sudden onset of unilateral deafness and vertigo. Pathological examination of the inner ear reveals hemorrhage into the perilymphatic space, with smaller focal hemorrhages in the endolymphatic space.[16] The vestibular and cochlear end organs, although morphologically intact, are rendered nonfunctional, apparently from altered fluid chemistry. A similar condition may follow from a blow to the head without the occurrence of a bony fracture (so-called **labyrinthine concussion**) (see p. 182).

Sudden-onset unilateral deafness and vertigo may result from hemorrhage into the inner ear in a patient with a bleeding diathesis such as leukemia.

Vertebrobasilar Transient Ischemic Attacks

Symptoms   Brief episodes of vertigo (minutes), usually in association with visual
                hallucinations, visual loss, diplopia, weakness, drop attacks, visceral sensations,
                headache, dysarthria, ataxia

Signs   Neurologic examination usually normal; may be signs of prior brain stem or
                cerebellar infarction, or both

Laboratory   *MRI:* Usually normal, may be old silent infarcts in occipital cortex or cerebellum
                Angiography: Usually atherosclerotic disease at vertebrobasilar junction region
                (Fig. 63)

Management   Antiplatelet drugs (aspirin 75–330 mg/day, ticlopidine 250 mg b.i.d)
                Anticoagulation for incapacitating, progressing symptoms and signs only: Begin
                heparin 5000 units IV bolus followed by continuous infusion of 1000 units per
                hour; dose is then titrated to keep the partial thromboplastin time at
                approximately 2.5 times control; after 3–4 days, warfarin is begun with an oral
                dose of 15 mg; the daily dose is adjusted (usually 5–15 mg) until the
                international normalized ratio (INR) is 2 to 3 times normal

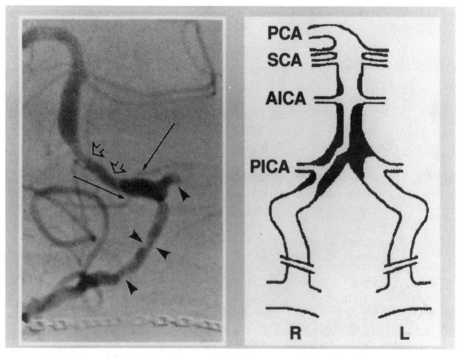

FIGURE 63 (*Left*) Cerebral angiogram in a patient with recurrent episodes of vertigo due to
vertebrobasilar insufficiency. Right vertebral artery injection (anterior posterior view). Arrowheads
show narrowing of the right vertebral artery and the left vertebral stump. (The left vertebral artery is
blocked.) Hollow arrows show basilar artery narrowing. The long, thin arrows point to the anterior
inferior cerebellar arteries. (*Right*) Schematic diagram of the anterior posterior view of the
vertebrobasilar system shown in the angiogram. AICA = anterior inferior cerebellar artery;
PCA = posterior cerebral artery; PICA = posterior inferior cerebellar artery; SCA = superior
cerebellar artery. (From Fife, TD, Baloh, RW, and Duckwiler, GR: Isolated dizziness in
vertebrobasilar insufficiency: Clinical features, angiography, and follow up. J Stroke Cerebrovasc Dis
4:4, 1994, with permission.)

Transient ischemia within the vertebrobasilar system is a common cause of a spontaneous attack of vertigo in older patients.[37] The vertigo is typically abrupt in onset, lasts several minutes, and is usually associated with other neurologic symptoms due to ischemia within the posterior circulation. Vertigo may be an isolated initial symptom of transient ischemia, or episodes of vertigo may be intermixed with more typical episodes with multiple symptoms, but long-standing recurrent episodes of vertigo without other symptoms would be highly atypical for transient ischemia within the vertebrobasilar system.[37,38]

The cause of vertebrobasilar TIAs is usually atherosclerosis of the subclavian, vertebral, and basilar arteries (Fig. 64). Vertigo is extremely common when the occlusive disease is localized to the distal vertebrals and vertebrobasilar junction region.[39] Other less

> *Episodic vertigo lasting several minutes in an older patient, sometimes alone but usually with accompanying neurologic symptoms, suggests transient ischemia in the vertebrobasilar system.*

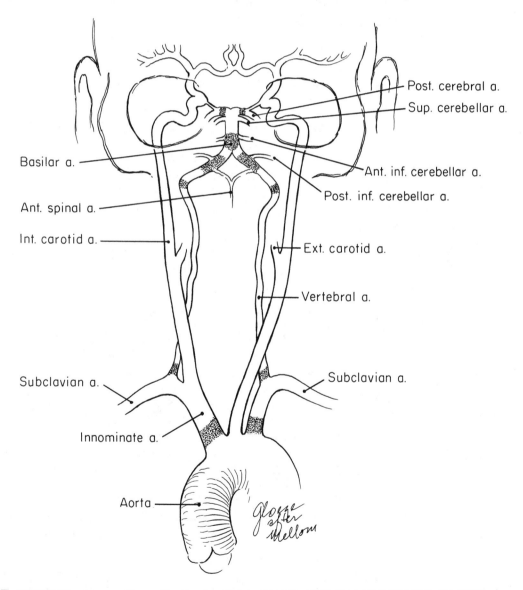

FIGURE 64 Areas with predilection for atherosclerosis within the vertebrobasilar circulation.

common causes of arterial occlusion include dissection, arteritis, emboli, polycythemia, thromboangiitis obliterans, and hypercoagulation syndromes.[40] Rarely, vertebrobasilar TIAs are precipitated by postural hypotension, Stokes-Adams attacks, or mechanical compression from cervical spondylosis. Cervical spondylosis is extremely common in older people, but documented cases of mechanical compression of the vertebral artery by neck turning or extension are rare. Most patients have multiple risk factors for atherosclerotic vascular disease, and often there is a prior history of myocardial infarction or occlusive peripheral vascular disease.

Lateral Medullary Infarction (Wallenberg's Syndrome)

Symptoms   Acute onset of vertigo, nausea, vomiting, imbalance, incoordination, hiccuping, facial pain, diplopia, dysphagia, dysphonia

Signs   (1) Ipsilateral Horner's syndrome; (2) ipsilateral paralysis of the palate, pharynx, and larynx; (3) ipsilateral loss of pain and temperature sensation on face; (4) ipsilateral dysmetria, dysrhythmia, and dysdiadochokinesia; (5) contralateral loss of pain and temperature sensation on body; (6) spontaneous nystagmus

Laboratory   *MRI:* Wedge of infarction in dorsolateral medulla (Fig. 65B), with or without infarction of posterior inferior cerebellum[41]
                Angiography: Occlusion of ipsilateral vertebral artery in most cases
                ENG: Spontaneous nystagmus may change direction with loss of fixation; lateropulsion of voluntary saccades; ipsilateral vestibular paresis to caloric stimulation

Management   Symptomatic treatment of vertigo (see Chapter 11)
                Antiplatelet drugs (aspirin or ticlopidine) to prevent future thrombotic episodes

If a patient's body and extremities seem to be pulled to one side, consider a lateral medullary infarction on that side.

The zone of infarction producing Wallenberg's syndrome consists of a wedge of the dorsolateral medulla just posterior to the olive (see Fig. 65). Although the syndrome is commonly known as that of the posterior inferior cerebellar artery (PICA), it usually results from occlusion of the ipsilateral vertebral artery and only rarely from the occlusion of the PICA itself.[42] Patients with Wallenberg's syndrome suffer a prominent motor disturbance that causes their body and extremities to deviate toward the side of the lesion as though pulled by a strong external force.[43] This so-called **lateropulsion** also affects the oculomotor system, causing excessively large voluntary and involuntary saccades directed toward the side of the lesion, whereas saccades away from the lesion are abnormally small.[44] Patients typically have an ocular tilt reaction (ipsilateral head tilt, skew deviation with the ipsilateral eye lower, and ocular torsion) (see Fig. 30). Even with their head

FIGURE 65   (*A*) Cross section of the medulla illustrating the zone of infarction with Wallenberg's syndrome (stippled area). (*B*) MRI of the posterior fossa (T$_2$-weighted, transverse section) demonstrating infarction of the right lateral medulla (arrow) in a patient with Wallenberg's syndrome.

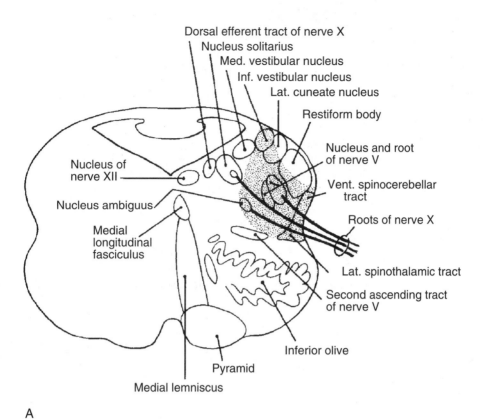

Dorsal efferent tract of nerve X
Nucleus solitarius
Med. vestibular nucleus
Inf. vestibular nucleus
Lat. cuneate nucleus
Restiform body
Nucleus and root of nerve V
Nucleus of nerve XII
Vent. spinocerebellar tract
Nucleus ambiguus
Roots of nerve X
Medial longitudinal fasciculus
Lat. spinothalamic tract
Second ascending tract of nerve V
Inferior olive
Pyramid
Medial lemniscus

A

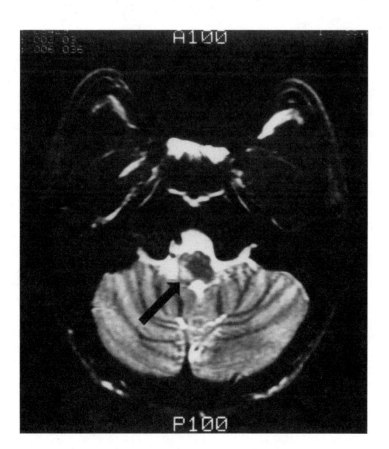

B

FIGURE 65 See facing page for legend.

Lateral Pontomedullary Infarction

Symptoms	Acute onset of vertigo, nausea and vomiting, unilateral hearing loss, tinnitus, facial paralysis, imbalance, and incoordination
Signs	(1) Ipsilateral hearing loss; (2) ipsilateral facial weakness; (3) ipsilateral loss of pain and temperature sensation on face; (4) ipsilateral dysmetria, dysrhythmia, and dysdiadochokinesia; (5) contralateral loss of pain and temperature sensation on body; (6) spontaneous nystagmus
Laboratory	*MRI:* Circular area of infarction in the dorsolateral pontomedullary region, with or without infarction of the anterior inferior cerebellum *Angiography:* Occlusion of ipsilateral vertebral artery in some cases *Audiometry:* Profound unilateral sensorineural deafness *ENG:* Spontaneous nystagmus that increases with loss of fixation, unilateral loss of caloric responses
Management	Symptomatic treatment of vertigo (see Chapter 11) Antiplatelet drugs (aspirin or ticlopidine) to prevent future thrombotic episodes

fixed in the true vertical, they perceive the environment as tilted opposite to the direction of the tilt reaction.

Ischemia in the distribution of the anterior inferior cerebellar artery (AICA) usually results in infarction of the dorsolateral pontomedullary region and the anterior inferior cerebellum.[45,46] Since the labyrinthine artery arises from the AICA in about 85% of cases, infarction of the membranous labyrinth is a common accompaniment. The AICA typically loops into the cerebellopontine angle, and not infrequently the loop enters the internal auditory canal, where it gives rise to the internal auditory artery. It also gives rise to one or more recurrent penetrating arteries that supply the lateral pontomedullary junction (Fig. 66). Occlusion within the AICA may lead to a sequential infarction in the lateral pons, as one recurrent penetrating artery after another is occluded. In some cases, facial paralysis is delayed for 1 to 2 days after the onset of infarction. Because both the labyrinth and the lateral brain stem are infarcted, the clinical syndrome has a characteristic combination of peripheral and central vestibular findings.

> *A combination of peripheral and central vestibular findings with unilateral hearing loss and facial paralysis may reflect a lateral pontomedullary infarction.*

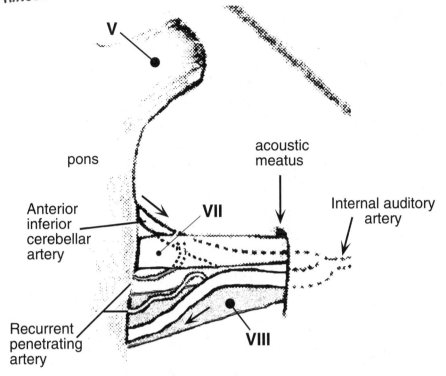

FIGURE 66 Anatomical features of the anteroinferior cerebellar artery (AICA) in the cerebellar pontine angle. The recurrent penetrating arteries supply the lateral pontomedullary junction. V = trigeminal nerve; VII = facial nerve; VIII = cochlear-vestibular nerve. Short arrows indicate the direction of blood flow. (Adapted form Oas, J and Baloh, RW. Vertigo and the anterior inferior cerebellar artery syndrome. Neurology 42:2274, 1992, with permission.)

Cerebellar Infarction

Symptoms   Acute-onset vertigo, nausea, and vomiting associated with severe imbalance and
                incoordination

Signs   Spontaneous or gaze-evoked nystagmus, truncal ataxia, dysrhythmia, and
                dysmetria of extremities

Laboratory   *MRI:* Infarction in territory of one of the cerebellar arteries (Fig. 67) or in the
                watershed areas between territories[47]
                ENG: Spontaneous nystagmus changes direction with change in gaze; dysmetria
                of voluntary saccades, impaired smooth pursuit, and optokinetic nystagmus

Management   Symptomatic treatment of vertigo (see Chapter 11)
                Close observation; may require surgical decompression if massive edema occurs
                Antiplatelet drugs (aspirin or ticlopidine) to prevent future thromboembolic events

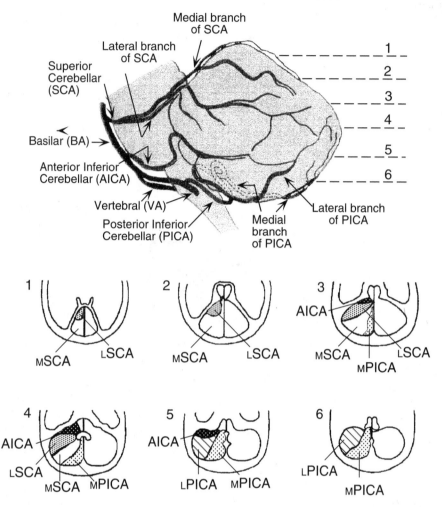

FIGURE 67 (*Top*) Branches of the three main cerebellar arteries. (*Bottom*) MRI horizontal axial sections from rostral to caudal (1–6), showing territory supplied by each branch. (Adapted from Amarenco, P: The spectrum of cerebellar infarctions. Neurology 41:973, 1991, with permission.)

When a patient appears to have a peripheral vestibular lesion but also shows cerebellar signs, the lesion may be a midline cerebellar infarction.

Atherosclerotic occlusion of the vertebrals and the PICA or AICA leads to a characteristic combination of brain stem and cerebellar infarction. However, **emboli** entering the posterior circulation often lead to infarction confined to the cerebellum, without brain stem involvement.[48] Infarction within the superior cerebellar artery territory is nearly always embolic. Infarction in the distribution of the medial cerebellar branch of the PICA can lead to a clinical presentation similar to that of a peripheral vestibular lesion.[49] The patient develops severe vertigo, nausea, and vomiting, along with imbalance but without associated brain stem symptoms. The key differential point is the finding on examination of cerebellar signs, including spontaneous nystagmus that changes direction with gaze and profound ataxia.[50] After a latent interval of

24 to 96 hours, some patients develop progressive brain stem dysfunction due to compression by a swollen cerebellum and hydrocephalus. A relentless progression to quadriplegia, coma, and death follows unless the compression is surgically relieved.

Cerebellar Hemorrhage

Symptoms   Acute-onset vertigo, nausea, and vomiting associated with headache and inability to stand

Signs   (1) Spontaneous or gaze-evoked nystagmus, (2) nuchal rigidity, (3) facial paralysis, (4) gaze paralysis, (5) marked truncal ataxia, (6) dysrhythmia and dysmetria of extremities, (7) bilateral small but reactive pupils

Laboratory   *MRI and CT:* Circumscribed lesion in cerebellum (hyperdense on CT); distortion of fourth ventricle, hydrocephalus, and brain stem compression common (Fig. 68)
                ENG: Spontaneous nystagmus changes direction with change in gaze; dysmetria of voluntary saccades, impaired smooth pursuit, and optokinetic nystagmus

Management   Surgical decompression usually required

Spontaneous intraparenchymal hemorrhage into the brain stem or cerebellum produces a dramatic clinical syndrome frequently progressing to loss of consciousness and death. The cause of hemorrhage is hypertensive vascular disease in approximately two thirds of patients. Anticoagulation therapy, cryptic arteriovenous malformations, and bleeding diatheses are also important etiological factors, whether alone or in combination with hypertension. Because of its potential reversibility, cerebellar hemorrhage deserves particular emphasis.[51] The initial symptoms of acute cerebellar hemorrhage are vertigo, nausea, vomiting, headache, and inability to stand or walk. As with cerebellar infarction, these symptoms might be confused with an acute peripheral vestibular lesion. Unlike cerebellar infarction, however, examination in the initial period usually reveals nuchal rigidity, prominent cerebellar signs, ipsilateral facial paralysis, and ipsilateral gaze paralysis. Pupils are often small bilaterally but reactive. Approximately 50% of patients lose consciousness within 24 hours of the initial symptoms, and 75% become comatose within 1 week of onset.[52] The condition is often fatal unless surgical decompression is performed. Midline cerebellar hemorrhage is particularly difficult to diagnose because it produces bilateral signs and generally runs a more fulminant course than lateralized hemorrhage. Such patients have profound ataxia, usually being unable to stand—a finding never associated with benign peripheral vestibular lesions.

Acute-onset vertigo, nausea, vomiting, and headache in a hypertensive patient, especially with the inability to stand, should prompt a search for a cerebellar hemorrhage, a serious but potentially reversible disorder.

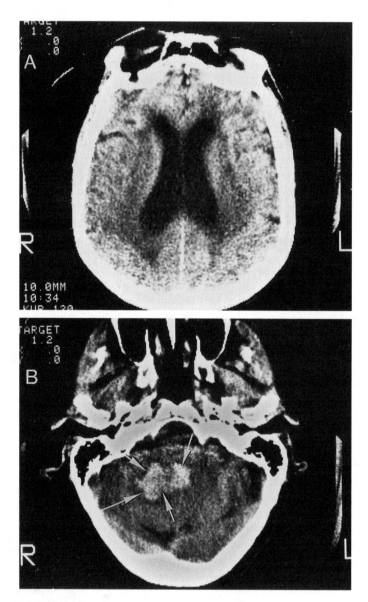

FIGURE 68   CT scans showing hydrocephalus (*A*) caused by cerebellar hemorrhage. (*B*) Arrows outline hemorrhage.

BENIGN POSITIONAL VERTIGO (CANALITHIASIS)

Benign positional vertigo (BPV) is not a disease but rather a syndrome that can be the sequela of several different inner ear diseases; in more than half the cases, no cause can be found.[53] Patients with BPV develop brief episodes of vertigo and nystagmus with position change, so that invariably some episodes occur in bed. The syndrome is important to recognize because in nearly all patients it can be cured with a simple bedside maneuver (explained later). The diagnosis is easily made at the bedside (see Fig. 29), so that extensive diagnostic procedures are not needed (see Pathological Nystagmus in Chapter 5). About half of the patients with BPV will have at least one recurrence after remission, and in some patients bouts of BPV are intermixed with variable periods of remission for many years. When a cause is found, it is most often either head trauma or a prior viral inner ear syndrome. Among patients in whom no cause can be found, females outnumber males by more than 2:1 and the peak age of onset is in the sixth decade.[54]

> *Benign positional vertigo (BPV) typically can be diagnosed and cured using bedside maneuvers.*

Benign Positional Vertigo — Posterior Canal Variant

Symptoms	Brief episodes of vertigo (usually <30 seconds) induced by turning over in bed, getting in and out of bed, bending down and straightening up, reaching for something on a high shelf ("top-shelf vertigo")
Signs	Torsional upbeat paroxysmal positioning nystagmus induced by rapid change from sitting to head-hanging position (see Fig. 29); usually fatigues with repeated positioning
Laboratory	*ENG:* Vestibular paresis to caloric stimulation in approximately one fourth of cases
Management	Particle repositioning maneuver (Fig. 69)

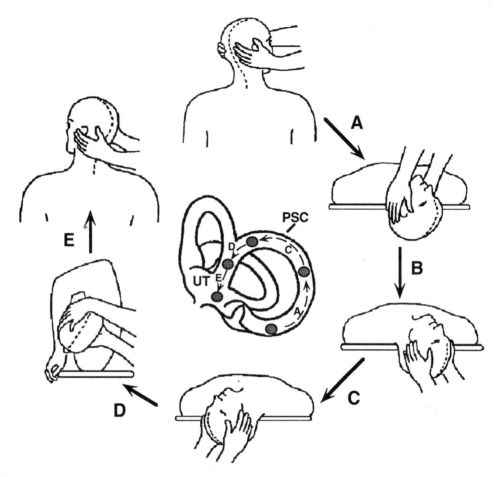

FIGURE 69   Treatment maneuver for benign positional vertigo affecting the right ear. The procedure can be reversed for treating the left ear. (*A*) The patient is seated upright, with the head facing the examiner, who is standing on the right. The patient should grasp the forearm of the examiner with both hands for stability. The patient is then moved into the supine position, allowing the head to extend just beyond the end of the examining table, with the right ear downward. this position is maintained until the nystagmus ceases. (*B*) The examiner moves to the head of the table, repositioning the hands as shown. (*C*) The head is rotated toward the left, stopping with the right ear upward. This position is maintained for 30 seconds. (*D*) The patient rolls onto the left side, while the examiner rotates the head leftward until the nose is directed toward the floor. This position is then held for 30 seconds. (*E*) The patient is lifted into the sitting position, now facing left. The entire sequence should be repeated until no nystagmus can be elicted. Labyrinth in the center shows the position of the debris before and after each position change as it moves around and out of the posterior semicircular canal (PSC) and into the utricle (UT). (Adapted from Foster, CA and Baloh, RW: Episodic vertigo. In: *Conn's Current Therapy.* Rakel, RE (ed). WB Saunders, Philadelphia, 1995, pp. 837–891 with permission.

> *Brief episodes of vertigo after turning over in bed or bending down and straightening up typify the posterior canal variant of BPV.*

The **posterior canal variant** is by far the most common type of BPV. A characteristic paroxysmal positioning nystagmus is consistent with the known excitatory connections of the posterior semicircular canal to the vertical oculomotor neurons.[53] Stimulation of the ampullary nerve from the posterior semicircular canal in animals produces identical nystagmus.[55] The typical features of BPV are explained by freely floating otoconial debris moving within the posterior semicircular canal under the influence of gravity (so-called **canalithiasis**).[56–58] With the patient sitting upright, a clot of calcium carbonate crystals forms at the most dependent portion of the posterior canal. Movement back and to the side in the plane of the posterior canal (as with the standard Dix-Hallpike positioning test) causes the clot to move in an ampullofugal direction, producing an ampullofugal displacement of the cupula as the clot moves within the narrow canal. Fatigability with repeated positioning is explained by dispersion of single particles from the clot, making the plunger less effective. During prolonged bed rest, the particles re-form into a clot, and the positional vertigo is reactivated. The induced vertigo and nystagmus are brief because once the clot reaches its lowest position in the canal with respect to the earth's surface, cupular elasticity returns the cupula to the primary position. Latency before onset of nystagmus is explained by the delay in setting the clot into motion.

Support for the posterior semicircular canal origin of BPV was provided by surgical procedures to section the ampullary nerve from the posterior semicircular canal or to block the posterior semicircular canal with a bony plug.[59,60] Both of these procedures are successful in curing intractable cases of BPV. In the process of exposing the membranous labyrinth of the posterior semicircular canal for the plugging operation, a chalky white substance was observed within the endolymph of the posterior canal.[60] This finding supported the canalithiasis theory and suggested that the debris is calcium carbonate crystals floating freely within the endolymph. Probably the most convincing argument for the canalithiasis theory is the dramatic response of the posterior canal variant of BPV to the positional maneuver designed to relocate the clot from the posterior canal into the utricle (Fig. 69).[58]

Benign Positional Vertigo — Horizontal Canal Variant

Symptoms	Brief episodes of vertigo (usually <60 seconds) induced by turning over in bed or when turning the head to the side while lying back in a chair
Signs	Direction-changing horizontal (geotropic) nystagmus induced by turning head to side while patient lies supine
Laboratory	*ENG:* Vestibular paresis to caloric stimulation in about one fourth of cases
Management	Particle repositioning maneuver: while lying supine, patient rotates toward the normal side in 90° steps (barbecue spit rotation)

Although rare compared with the posterior canal variant of BPV, the **horizontal canal variant** is important to recognize because it has features that have been attributed to central nervous system lesions.[61–63] The clinical history is similar to that of the posterior canal variant, but there are important differences. With both syndromes, positional vertigo occurs in bed, particularly

The horizontal canal variant of BPV, much less common than the posterior canal variant, can cause vertigo when patients simply turn their head, especially while leaning back.

when patients turn over from one side to the other. Patients with the horizontal canal variant, however, may develop vertigo when turning the head to the side while leaning back in a chair or even occasionally when turning the head to the side while standing or walking. Remissions and exacerbations occur with both types of BPV, but exacerbations are typically shorter with the horizontal canal variant than with the posterior canal variant.[62,63] Interestingly, the horizontal canal variant can occur after patients with the posterior canal variant are treated with the particle repositioning maneuver.[64] Presumably the debris leaves the posterior canal and enters the horizontal canal, where it causes symptoms under the influence of gravity.

The horizontal canal variant of BPV is due to accumulation of debris in the long arm of the horizontal semicircular canal, analogous to the mechanism of the posterior canal variant (Fig. 70).[63] When the head is rapidly turned to the abnormal side, the debris is accelerated downward in the canal. The movement of the clot within the canal causes an ampullopetal deviation of the cupula and a burst of nystagmus beating toward the ground. When the clot stops moving, elasticity returns the cupula to the primary position. Once the free-floating clot moves to the bottom of the canal in the lateral position, returning to the supine position moves the clot back to the original position and causes a burst of nystagmus in the opposite direction. Rotation of the head to the normal side causes the clot to move toward the utricle and produces an ampullofugal displacement of the cupula and nystagmus beating toward the ground. For the particle repositioning maneuver, the patient rotates the head toward the normal side in 90° steps to move the debris from the canal into the utricle.[53]

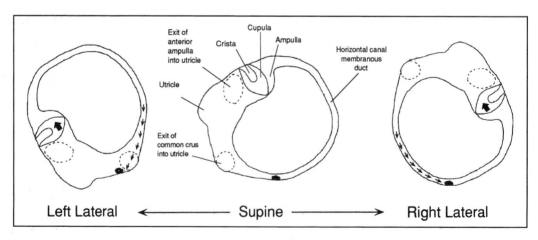

FIGURE 70   Mechanism of the horizontal canal variant of BPV involving the right ear. The position of the utricle and ampulla relative to the head was derived from CT scans of normal temporal bones with cuts through the horizontal semicircular canals. With the head in the right lateral position, the debris moves toward the cupula (small arrows), causing an ampullopetal deviation (large arrow) and right-beating nystagmus. The reverse occurs with the head in the left lateral position. (From Baloh, RW, Jacobson, K, and Honrubia, V: Horizontal semicircular canal variant of benign positional vertigo. Neurology 43:2542, 1993, with permission.)

MÉNIÈRE'S DISEASE (ENDOLYMPHATIC HYDROPS)

Symptoms   Fluctuating hearing loss, tinnitus, ear fullness, and vertigo; may have sudden falling episodes (otolithic crises)

Signs   Hearing loss that increases during attacks; spontaneous nystagmus and gait unsteadiness during attacks

Laboratory   *Audiometry:* Low-frequency sensorineural hearing loss that increases during attacks (see Fig. 39C); recruitment usually present
                  Electrocochleography: Ratio of summating potential to action potential > 0.5
                  ENG: Spontaneous or positional nystagmus most prominent with eyes closed or open in darkness; vestibular paresis or directional preponderance to caloric stimulation

Management   *Medical:* (1) To prevent attacks, sodium restriction and diuretic (begin with 1 g Na^+ per day and hydroclorothiazide 50 mg or acetazolamide 250 mg per day[65]; (2) antivertiginous medication during attack (see Chapter 11)
                  Surgical: (1) Endolymphatic sac operations (controversial because of conflicting evidence of efficacy); (2) destructive procedures (transtympanic gentamicin, labyrinthectomy, or vestibular nerve section) for patients with disabling vertigo and unilateral severe hearing loss who do not respond to medical treatment[66,67]

Ménière's disease is characterized by fluctuating hearing loss and tinnitus, episodic vertigo, and a sensation of fullness or pressure in the ear.[68] Variations from this classic picture occur, particularly in the early stages of the disease process; the diagnosis remains uncertain without the combination of fluctuating hearing loss and vertigo. Rarely, isolated episodes of vertigo or hearing loss will precede the characteristic combination of symptoms by months and possibly even years. Although so-called **vestibular Ménière's** and **cochlear Ménière's** have been proposed as variations of the classic disease, clinical pathological correlation of isolated vestibular and auditory disorders with selective endolymphatic hydrops of the vestibular and auditory labyrinth is lacking. Speculation regarding the relationship between migraine and Ménière's disease dates back to the initial description by Ménière.[69] Probably most cases of vestibular Ménière's disease are due to migraine. Whether migraine leads to damage of the inner ear and ultimate development of endolymphatic hydrops or whether the basic biochemical defect with migraine can mimic Ménière's disease is unknown.

So-called **delayed endolymphatic hydrops** develops in an ear that has been damaged years before, usually by a viral or bacterial infection.[16,70] With this disorder, the patient reports a long history of hearing loss since early childhood, followed many year later by typical symptoms and signs of Ménière's disease. If the hearing loss is profound, as it often is, the episodic vertigo will not be ac-

A diagnosis of Ménière's disease depends upon a combination of fluctuating hearing loss and episodic vertigo.

companied by fluctuating hearing levels and tinnitus. Pathological studies in such patients suggest that delayed endolymphatic hydrops results from damage to the resorptive mechanism of the inner ear from the initial insult; it eventually leads to an imbalance between secretion and resorption of endolymph. Delayed endolymphatic hydrops can be unilateral or bilateral, depending on the extent of the damage at the time of the original insult.

The principal pathological finding in patients with Ménière's disease is an increase in the volume of endolymph, associated with distention of the entire endolymphatic system (Fig. 71).[16] The episodes of hearing loss and vertigo may be caused by ruptures in the membranes separating endolymph from perilymph, producing a sudden increase in potassium concentration in the perilymph. Another possible explanation for the fluctuating symptoms is mechanical deformation of the end organ that is reversible as the endolymphatic pressure decreases. The dramatic sudden falling attacks originally described by Tumarkin are probably due to sudden deformation or displacement of one of the otolith organs.[71]

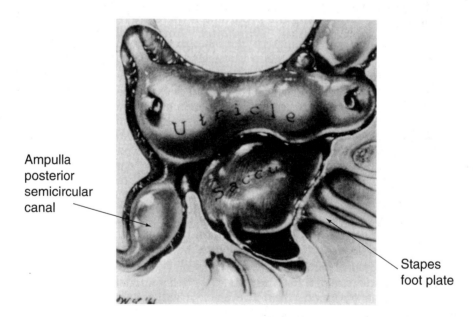

Ampulla posterior semicircular canal

Stapes foot plate

FIGURE 71   Endolymphatic hydrops. The volume of endolymph is increased, leading to distention of the entire endolymphatic system. Note that the dilated saccular wall makes contact with the stapes footplate.

AUTOIMMUNE INNER EAR DISEASE

Symptoms	Fluctuating, sometimes slowly progressive hearing loss; tinnitus; episodic vertigo; progresses from unilateral to bilateral, may be associated with systemic symptoms; steroid responsive
Signs	Spontaneous nystagmus, hearing loss; may be accompanied by interstitial keratitis, arthritis, rash, and so forth
Laboratory	*ENG:* Decreased caloric response *Audiometry:* Sensorineural hearing loss May be features of systemic vasculitis; lymphocyte transformation; anticochlear antibodies[72,73]
Management	High-dose steroids (60–100 mg prednisone, 12–16 mg dexamethasone) for 10 days, then taper; consider cytotoxic drugs or plasmapheresis if symptoms recur or steroids cause adverse effects[74]

Autoimmune inner ear disease is an uncommon but important cause of progressive, bilateral loss of auditory and vestibular function.[72,75] Inner ear dysfunction may begin on one side, but invariably it progresses to involve both sides, leading to profound deafness and vestibular loss if treatment is not instituted. Three characteristic clinical profiles have been recognized:

1. Inner ear involvement as part of a systemic autoimmune disorder (e.g., polyarteritis, rheumatoid arthritis, ulcerative colitis)
2. Inner ear involvement plus interstitial keratitis (**Cogan's syndrome**) (see Fig. 61)
3. Isolated inner ear involvement

Often patients will move from one category to another, with the most typical progression being from 3 or 2 to 1. Clinical symptoms often begin with fluctuating hearing loss, ear pressure, and tinnitus, along with vertigo, suggesting Ménière's disease. Unlike Ménière's disease, however, these symptoms rapidly progress over weeks to months to involve the opposite ear. Occasionally there is a slow, progressive bilateral sensorineural hearing loss accompanied by a progressive bilateral loss of vestibular function.

The blood-labyrinth barrier is analogous to the blood-brain barrier with respect to immunoglobulin equilibrium, and the inner ear can respond to an antigen challenge just as the brain can.[74] Probably both cell-mediated and humoral immune pathways are involved in the production of autoimmune inner ear disease. As many as two thirds of these patients have antibodies directed against cochlear antigens.[72,73] The mechanism by which these antibodies lead to inner ear damage is yet to be determined.

Symptoms of autoimmune inner ear disease may resemble Ménière's disease at first, but they rapidly progress to involve the opposite ear.

MIGRAINE (BENIGN RECURRENT VERTIGO)

Symptoms   Headache (Table 19), visual aura, episodic vertigo (often separate from headaches), motion sickness

Signs   Normal examination

Laboratory   *ENG:* Decreased caloric response in approximately 20% of patients
                  MRI: Small T_2-intense lesions

Management   (Of vertigo and motion sickness)
                  Prophylactic: β-Blockers (propranolol 120–240 mg/day), calcium channel blockers (verapamil 120–240 mg/day), tricyclic amines (nortriptyline 75–150 mg/day)
                  Symptomatic: Phenergan 25 mg and/or metoclopramide 10 mg at first symptom and then q 4 h as needed

About a quarter of patients with migraine experience vertigo, sometimes without headache.

Vertigo is a common symptom with migraine, occurring in about one quarter of patients.[76] It can vary in duration from minutes to hours and can occur without headache. With **basilar migraine**, vertigo is associated with other posterior fossa symptoms such as ataxia, dysarthria, and visual phenomena.[77] Basilar migraine is most commonly seen in adolescent girls, often occurring in association with their menstrual periods, but it can occur at any age. So-called **benign paroxysmal vertigo of childhood** and **benign recurrent vertigo of adulthood** nearly always turn out to be migraine.[33] Patients with these migraine equivalents may or may not develop typical migraine headaches at another time in their life.

The mechanism for vertigo associated with migraine is poorly understood. Vasoconstriction involving the internal auditory artery could explain some symptoms, but one would expect a higher incidence of associated hearing loss if this were the typical

---

Table 19 International Headache Society (IHS) Diagnostic Criteria for Migraine Headaches

A. At least 5 attacks fulfilling B–D
B. Headache lasts 4–72 hours (untreated)
C. Headache has at least two of the following features:
    1. Unilateral
    2. Pulsating
    3. Moderate or severe (inhibits or prohibits daily activities)
    4. Aggravated by walking, stairs, or similar physical activities
D. During headache at least one of the following:
    1. Nausea and vomiting
    2. Photophobia and phonophobia
E. Other causes of headache have been ruled out

Adapted from Olesen J: Headache Classification Committee of the International Headache Society: Classification and diagnostic criteria for headache disorders, cranial neuralgias and facial pain. Cephalalgia 8 (Suppl 7):1, 1988.

mechanism for the vertigo.[78] Although hearing loss does occur with migraine, it is infrequent compared with the incidence of vertigo. Phonophobia and tinnitus are more common than hearing loss, with phonophobia being more prominent during the period of severe headaches.[79] An association between migraine and Ménière's disease, initially suggested by Ménière himself, complicates the matter further.[80] Numerous case reports describe migraine and Ménière's attacks occurring in the same patient. Typically the patient has migraine for many years before developing symptoms and signs of Ménière's disease. There is often correspondence in the laterality of the hearing loss and migrainous headache and in the occurrence of attacks of vertigo. More than one half of patients with migraine experience severe sensitivity to motion, with frequent bouts of motion sickness.[33] The mechanism of this sensitivity to motion with migraine is unknown.

Clinicians have long suspected a genetic cause for migraine; there is a positive family history in most cases. Familial aggregation studies suggest a combination of genetic and environmental factors in the production of migraine. An uncommon variety with a clear autosomal dominant mode of inheritance is **hemiplegic migraine**. Recently several families with hemiplegic migraine were found to have a missense mutation in a calcium channel gene located on chromosome 19p.[81] Interestingly, when families with hemiplegic migraine are carefully investigated, more than 50% of affected members meet the clinical criteria for basilar migraine, suggesting that these two disorders may be allelic to the same gene.[82]

TUMORS

Tumors of the Middle Ear and the Temporal Bone

Symptoms	Ear fullness and pain, hearing loss, otorrhea, mastoid swelling, facial paralysis, rarely vertigo
Signs	Tumor may be visible after erosion into the external auditory canal, through the mastoid cortex into the skin, or behind the tympanic membrane
Laboratory	*Audiometry:* Conductive hearing loss *Imaging:* CT is best for determining extent of bony involvement and MRI is most useful for determining soft tissue extent; angiography and jugular venography can help identify a glomus body tumor
Management	Surgical removal where possible, subtotal resection followed by irradiation in others

A wide variety of benign and malignant tumors involve the middle ear and the temporal bone. Tumors involving the middle ear produce symptoms of fullness or conductive hearing loss early, whereas tumors in the temporal bone outside the middle ear

Tumors of the middle ear cause early conductive hearing loss or fullness, but tumors in the temporal bone may become quite large without producing symptoms.

can become quite large without producing symptoms. The tumor may not become apparent until it erodes into the external auditory canal or through the mastoid cortex into the skin. Anterior extension into the cavernous sinus produces ophthalmoplegia from involvement of nerves III, IV, and VI. Malignant tumors in this region tend to spread locally to the regional lymph nodes; distant metastasis is unusual. Ultimately the tumor can be seen in the nasopharynx, middle ear, or neck.

Squamous cell carcinoma is the most frequent histologic type of malignant tumor involving the middle ear and mastoid.[83] It typically arises from epidermal cells in the auricle and external auditory canal or the middle ear and mastoid (Fig. 72). Prognosis is good for tumors confined to the auricle and external canal but not for those invading the middle ear and mastoid.[84] Rhabdomyosarcoma is the most common malignant tumor of the middle ear in children. The initial symptom is often facial paralysis, which may be mistakenly diagnosed as idiopathic Bell's palsy. Metastatic tumor involvement of the temporal bone is common with several different tumor types, but because of the endochondral layer's resistance, neoplasms rarely invade the bony labyrinth.[16]

Glomus body tumors are the most common tumor of the middle ear and the second most common tumor of the temporal bone, next to schwannomas.[85] The most common tumor sites are the glomus jugulare (jugular bulb), glomus tympanicum (middle ear), and glomus vagale (along the course of the vagus nerve). Glomus vagale and jugulare tumors often involve the labyrinth and the cranial nerves, whereas glomus tympanicum tumors usually produce only local symptoms such as conductive hearing loss, pulsatile tinnitus, and rhinorrhea, which occur because of the tumor bulk in the middle ear.

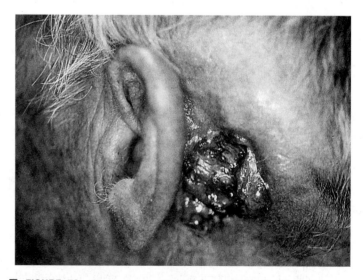

FIGURE 72 Squamous cell carcinoma originating from epidermal cells behind the auricle. (Courtesy Akira Ishiyama, M.D., Head and Neck Surgery, UCLA.)

Tumors of the Cerebellopontine Angle

Symptoms	Slowly progressive unilateral hearing loss, tinnitus, disequilibrium; infrequent vertigo (in approximately 10–20% of cases)
Signs	Unilateral hearing loss, ipsilateral facial weakness, other lower cranial nerve findings in late stages[86]
Laboratory	*Audiometry:* Unilateral sensorineural hearing loss associated with poor speech discrimination, abnormal BAER (only wave I present, prolonged I–V interval) *ENG:* Ipsilateral vestibular paresis to bithermal caloric stimulation *Imaging:* MRI with contrast is the procedure of choice (Fig. 73); it can identify small tumors confined to the internal auditory canal, tumors that are missed with CT scanning; CT scanning may be of some help for identifying a bony erosion and/or calcification within tumors
Management	Surgical removal in most cases; small acoustic neuromas in elderly patients may be followed with serial imaging, since the tumor may remain confined to the internal auditory canal for years[87]

Tumors arising in the narrow confines of the internal auditory canal typically produce a gradual compression of cranial nerves VII and VIII.[87] Sensorineural hearing loss, tinnitus, and facial paresis evolve insidiously, usually over months to years. Vertigo is uncommon with such lesions because the nervous system is able to adapt to the gradual loss of vestibular function. Lesions within the cerebellopontine (C-P) angle produce a similar slowly progressive compression of cranial nerves VII and VIII, although tumors arising in the angle can grow to a much larger size before critical compression occurs. Most often, tumors begin in the internal auditory canal and grow outward into the C-P angle, following the path of least resistance. Next to nerves VII and VIII, nerve V is most commonly involved with C-P angle tumors, causing ipsilateral facial numbness. In later stages of progression, involvement of nerves VI, IX, and X may give rise to diplopia, dysphonia, and dysphagia. Compression of the brain stem and cerebellum causes ipsilateral gaze dysfunction and dysmetria of the extremities.

Acoustic neuromas are by far the most common C-P angle tumor, accounting for more than 90% of tumors in this region.[88] A more appropriate name would be "vestibular schwannoma," since more than 90% of these tumors arise from Schwann cells of the vestibular nerve.[33] Meningiomas are the next most common tumor of the C-P angle, followed by epidermoid cysts and facial-nerve schwannomas.[88] Cholesterol granulomas arise in the pneumatized spaces of the temporal bone and can expand to compress the structures in the C-P angle.[89] It is an important lesion to recognize because the surgical management is quite different from that of tumors in the C-P angle. Detailed audiometric testing followed by neuroimaging with MRI will usually lead to a definitive diagnosis (Fig. 74).

Insidiously evolving unilateral sensorineural hearing loss, tinnitus, and facial paresis may signal a tumor in the internal auditory canal growing into the cerebellopontine angle.

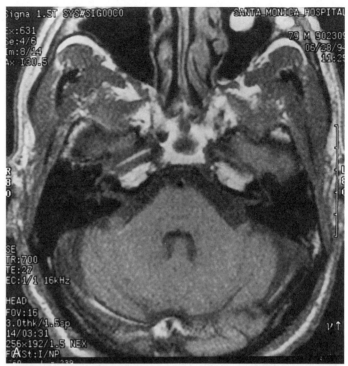

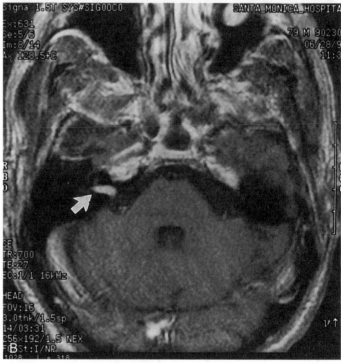

FIGURE 73 Magnetic resonance images (MRIs) (*A*) before and (*B*) after contrast, showing a small acoustic neuroma confined to the right internal auditory canal (arrow). T$_1$-weighted, transverse sections.

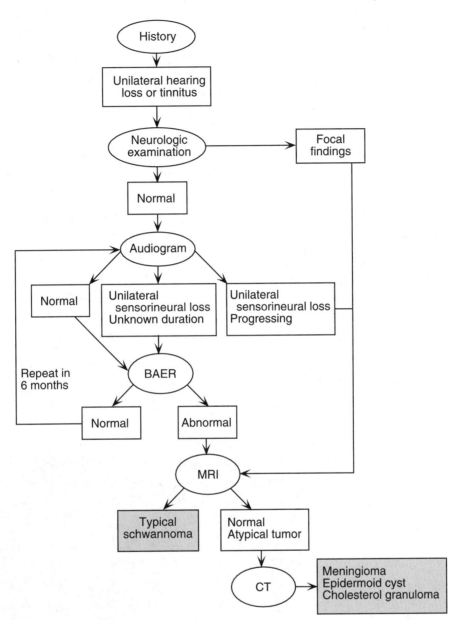

FIGURE 74 Algorithm for diagnosis of tumors of the cerebellopontine angle. BAER = brain stem auditory evoked response; CT = computerized tomography; MRI = magnetic resonance imaging. (Adapted from Baloh, RW and Honrubia, V: *Clinical Neurophysiology of the Vestibular System*, ed. 2. F. A. Davis, Philadelphia, 1990, p. 238, with permission.)

Tumors of the Posterior Fossa

Symptoms

Brain stem tumors: Vestibular and cochlear symptoms in >50% of cases; relentless progressive involvement of one brain stem center after another

Cerebellar tumors: Positional vertigo, vomiting, headache, and gait imbalance

Signs

Brain stem tumors: Combination of long tract signs, cranial nerve deficits, and ataxia

Cerebellar tumors: Central positional nystagmus, papilledema, ataxia; may be relatively silent until they become large enough to obstruct CSF circulation or compress the brain stem

Laboratory

Imaging: MRI is the diagnostic procedure of choice for identifying brain stem and cerebellar tumors (Fig. 75)[90]; CT can complement MRI by helping differentiate between tumor and associated edema

Audiometry: Hearing for pure tones is usually normal with brain stem tumors but abnormalities on BAER are common

ENG: Central types of spontaneous and positional nystagmus are common; abnormalities of smooth pursuit, saccades, and visuovestibular interaction

Management

When possible, biopsy and surgical resection of the tumor; radiation therapy when the tumor is nonresectable (medulloblastomas are particularly sensitive to radiation therapy)

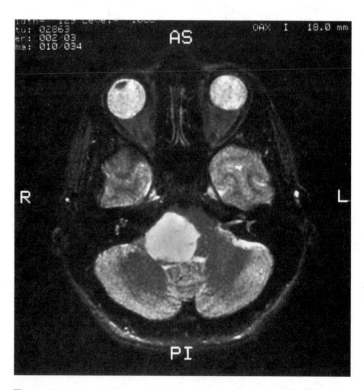

FIGURE 75   MRI (T_2-weighted) showing a brain stem glioma involving the root entry zone of the right eighth nerve.

Gliomas of the brain stem usually grow slowly and infiltrate the brain stem nuclei and fiber tracts, producing multiple symptoms and signs.[91] Tumors arising in the fourth ventricular region compress the vestibular nuclei and produce multiple vestibular symptoms. Medulloblastomas, occurring primarily in children and adolescents, are rapidly growing, highly cellular tumors that arise in the posterior midline or vermis of the cerebellum and invade the fourth ventricle and adjacent cerebellar hemispheres. Vertigo and disequilibrium are common initial complaints.[92] Gliomas of the cerebellum may be relatively silent until they become large enough to obstruct CSF circulation or compress the brain stem. As with medulloblastoma, positional vertigo is occasionally the initial symptom of a cerebellar glioma.[93,94] The associated paroxysmal positional nystagmus is central in type because it is vertical, induced in several positions, and nonfatigable. Other tumors that produce identical symptoms and signs include teratomas, hemangiomas, and hemangioblastomas.

> *Positional vertigo is occasionally the initial symptom of a cerebellar glioma or medulloblastoma; it may be associated with positional nystagmus of the central type.*

TRAUMA

Otitic Barotrauma

Symptoms	Sudden, severe ear pain during descent from high altitude or during ascent from underwater diving
Signs	Hyperemia of tympanic membrane, sometimes with fluid in middle ear, hearing loss on same side
Laboratory	*Audiometry:* Conductive hearing loss, restricted or flat tympanogram
Management	Usually spontaneously remits within several hours; if hearing loss persists, may require exploration of middle ear to rule out labyrinthine window rupture

Otitic barotrauma (aero-otitis) is a traumatic inflammatory disorder of the middle ear caused by sudden, severe negative pressure in the pneumatized spaces of the temporal bone.[16] The intense negative pressure causes medial displacement and stretching of the tympanic membrane, hyperemia and edema, and ecchymosis of the membranes of the middle ear followed by transudation of fluid, which may become sanguinous in severe cases. The main symptom is excruciating pain in the ear that gradually subsides over a period of hours. Occasionally there is an associated conductive hearing loss due to damage of the tympanic membrane and ossicular chain. Rarely, if there is rupture of the labyrinthine windows, there may be vertigo and sensorineural hearing loss.[95] Otitic barotrauma typically occurs during descent from high altitude or during ascent from underwater diving. It is caused by failure of the eustachian tube to open enough to permit the equalization of middle ear pressure.

Perilymph Fistula

Symptoms	"Popping" sound in ear, sudden-onset hearing loss, tinnitus, and vertigo associated with head trauma, barotrauma, cough, sneeze, straining, exercise, cholesteatoma, past ear surgery, congenital malformation
Signs	May be positive fistula sign: vertigo and nystagmus induced by pressure change in external canal or with coughing or straining
Laboratory	*ENG:* Decreased caloric response *Audiometry:* Sensorineural hearing loss *CT/MRI:* May show chronic otomastoiditis, cholesteatoma, malformed inner ear
Management	Bed rest, elevated head, symptomatic treatment, avoid straining Explore ear if symptoms persist or if clear relationship to trauma[96]

A perilymph fistula, often the result of a sudden pressure change, can have remarkably variable symptoms and signs.

A perilymph fistula results from disruption of the lining membranes of the labyrinth, usually at the oval or round windows. The symptoms and signs are remarkably variable; a perilymph fistula must be considered in the differential diagnosis of sudden hearing loss, recurrent vestibulopathy, Ménière's syndrome, congenital sensorineural hearing loss, posttraumatic hearing loss and vertigo, and stapedectomy failure.[96]

The cause of perilymph fistula is obvious when there is a disruption of the otic capsule or a tear in the membranous labyrinth associated with trauma, surgery, or infection (see Fig. 55); spontaneous fistulae are more difficult to explain. A sudden negative or positive pressure change in the middle ear from violent nose blowing, sneezing, or barotrauma, or a sudden increase in CSF pressure associated with lifting, straining, coughing, or vigorous activity could lead to rupture of the round window (Fig. 76).[97] In the latter case, the change in CSF pressure is transmitted to the inner ear by the cochlear aqueduct, internal auditory canal, or both. Perilymph fistulae may also be associated with developmental abnormalities of the middle ear and otic capsule, such as defects in the stapes footplate or other malformations of the stapedial arch.

How leakage of perilymph leads to fluctuating vestibular and auditory symptoms is unclear. Removal of the round window in animals has relatively little effect on cochlear function, and the perilymphatic space is routinely entered during stapedectomy surgery, usually without sequela. The cochleosacculotomy operation for Ménière's disease produces a round window membrane rupture, yet the incidence of postoperative sensorineural hearing loss is low (less than 25%).[98] Although the sensorineural hearing loss associated with perilymph fistulae is usually not reversible, patients occasionally have been reported to have dramatic recovery of hearing years after the onset of hearing loss.[33]

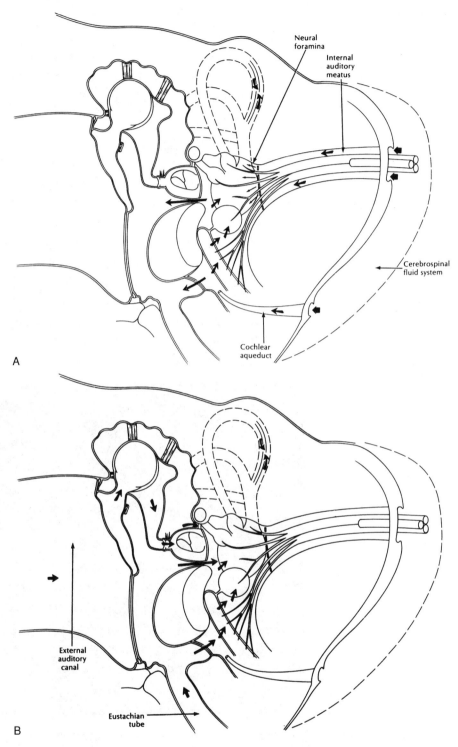

FIGURE 76 Causes of labyrinthine membrane ruptures. (*A*) Explosive forces from cerebrospinal fluid via the cochlear aqueduct or internal auditory canal; and (*B*) implosive forces from the middle ear, eustachian tube, and external ear. (From Goodhill, V: Sudden sensorineural deafness. Proc Roy Soc Med 69:565–572, 1976, with permission.)

Labyrinthine Concussion

Symptoms	Onset of vertigo, hearing loss, or both after a blow to the head (usually resulting in loss of consciousness); in some cases onset may be delayed for several days
Signs	Unilateral hearing loss; spontaneous nystagmus; usually normal external canal and tympanic membrane; may be blood, CSF, or both in external or middle ear if associated temporal bone fracture
Laboratory	*Audiometry:* Profound unilateral sensorineural hearing loss *ENG:* Spontaneous nystagmus most prominent with eyes closed or opened in darkness; decreased or absent caloric response on side of hearing loss *CT:* Usually normal, may be associated temporal bone fracture (Fig. 77)
Management	Symptomatic treatment of vertigo (see Chapter 11)

Labyrinthine concussion causing vertigo, hearing loss, and tinnitus often follows a blow to the head that does not result in temporal bone fracture.[99] Although protected by a bony capsule, the delicate labyrinthine membranes are susceptible to blunt trauma.[16] Blows to the occipital or mastoid regions are particularly likely to

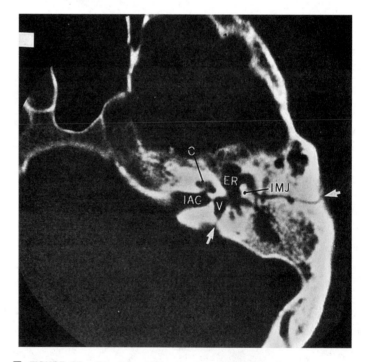

FIGURE 77   CT scans of the temporal bone showing longitudinal and transverse fractures in the same patient (arrows). The longitudinal fracture crosses the middle ear, disrupting the ossicular chain, while the transverse fracture enters the vestibule, damaging the membranous labyrinth. C = cochlea; ER = epitympanic recess; IAC = internal auditory canal; IMJ = incudomalleal joint; V = vestibule. (Courtesy William Hanafee, M.D., and Sven Larsen, M.D., Radiology, UCLA.)

produce labyrinthine damage. Paradoxically, a blow that does not fracture the skull may produce more labyrinthine damage than one in which the forces are absorbed by an actual break in the bones. The absence of associated brain stem symptoms and signs and the usual rapid improvement in symptoms following injury support a peripheral localization of most lesions.

Sudden deafness following a blow to the head, with or without associated vestibular symptoms, is often partially or completely reversible. It is probably caused by intense acoustic stimulation from pressure waves created by the blow that are transmitted through the bones to the cochlea just as pressure waves are transmitted from air through the conduction mechanism.[100] Supporting this suggestion, the pathological changes in the cochlea produced by experimental head blows in animals are similar to those produced by intense airborne sound stimuli.[101] These changes consist of degeneration of hair cells and cochlear neurons in the middle turns of the cochlea. Pure tone hearing loss is usually most pronounced at 4000 to 8000 Hz.

> *A blow to the head may damage delicate labyrinthine membranes, causing vertigo or hearing loss.*

Noise-Induced Hearing Loss

Symptoms	Gradual bilateral hearing loss and tinnitus with long-standing noise exposure; may be temporary threshold shift with brief exposure to intense sound (e.g., rock concert)
Signs	Bilateral high-frequency hearing loss
Laboratory	*Audiometry:* Bilateral sensorineural hearing loss with characteristic notch at 4000 Hz (see Fig. 39A)
Management	Remove from exposure to loud noise *Prevention:* Carefully monitor hearing levels in subjects at risk (e.g., workers in heavy industry), use ear plugs, control noise level

Noise-induced hearing loss is extremely common in our industrialized society. The loss almost always begins at 4000 Hz and does not affect speech discrimination until late in the disease process.[102] With only a brief exposure to loud noise (hours to days), there may be only a temporary threshold shift, but with continued exposure, permanent injury begins. Damage to sensory cells is often confined to a small area at the base of the cochlea, centering around the area sensing 4000 Hz.[16]

Two main theories explain the remarkable tendency for noise-induced injuries to involve this 8- to 10-mm region at the base of the cochlea.[16] The mechanical view holds that strong destructive forces develop owing to a "jet effect" at this particular region. The vascular theory maintains that this region is especially vulnerable to ischemia because it is at the juncture of the main cochlear artery and the cochlear ramus artery. Pathological studies in patients with typical noise-induced hearing loss document a loss of hair cells 5 to 10 mm from the base of the cochlea.[16] Electron microscope studies have re-

> *Bilateral sensorineural hearing loss caused by continued exposure to loud noise almost always begins at 4000 Hz.*

vealed a characteristic progression of changes in the hair cells of animals exposed to loud noise. Initially, blebs form on the surface of the hair cells, followed by vesiculation and vacuolization of the smooth endoplasmic reticulum, accumulation of lysosomal granules in the subcuticular region, deformation of the cuticular plate, and, finally, cell rupture and lysis (Fig. 78).

OTOTOXICITY

Symptoms	Bilateral sensorineural hearing loss and/or disequilibrium with oscillopsia
Signs	Decreased hearing, bilateral positive head thrust test, decreased dynamic visual acuity, gait unsteadiness, positive Romberg test
Laboratory	*Audiology:* Sensorineural hearing loss beginning in the high frequencies and progressing to a flat 60 to 70-dB loss across all frequencies *ENG:* Decreased caloric response bilaterally and decreased gain on rotational testing
Management	*Key to management is prevention:* Kidney function should be assessed and patients with abnormal kidney function should be carefully monitored; question patients regularly to identify early symptoms of auditory or vestibular loss Vestibular rehabilitation is useful for helping patients adapt to bilateral vestibular loss

To prevent auditory and vestibular damage, physicians must be aware of the ototoxic potential of drugs, especially for patients with renal impairment.

Patients who receive ototoxic drugs are often bedridden and suffer from multiple symptoms of systemic illness, so additional symptoms of auditory and vestibular dysfunction may be easily overlooked. Vestibular symptoms are particularly difficult to identify in this setting. Only after the patient begins to recover do the devastating effects of vestibular loss become apparent. By this time, the damage is irreversible. If ototoxicity is to be prevented, the examining physician must be keenly aware of the potential auditory and vestibular toxicity of any drug that is used.

Each of the aminoglycoside drugs can cause both auditory and vestibular damage, but gentamicin is relatively specific for the vestibular system, whereas kanamycin, tobramycin, and amikacin produce more damage to the auditory system.[103,104] The newer aminoglycosides dibekacin and netilmicin are overall less ototoxic than the older aminoglycosides.[105] The pharmacological and biochemical characteristics are similar for all of the aminoglycoside antibiotics.[106] They are excreted almost exclusively by glomerular filtration; they are not metabolized. Patients with renal impairment cannot excrete the drugs, so they accumulate in the blood and inner ear tissues. The ototoxicity of the aminoglycosides has been shown convincingly to be due to hair cell damage in the inner ear (Fig. 79). Unlike penicillin and other common antibiotics, aminoglycosides are concentrated in the perilymph and endolymph.[107]

The earliest effect of vestibulotoxic compounds such as streptomycin and gentamicin is a selective destruction of type I hair cells in

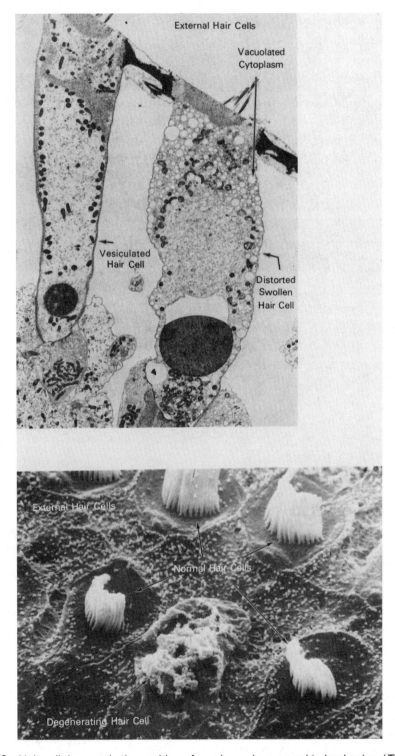

FIGURE 78 Hair cell damage in the cochlea of a guinea pig exposed to loud noise. (*Top*) Transmission electron microscopic section showing vesiculation and vacuolization of the endoplasmic reticulum of the external hair cells. (*Bottom*) Scanning electron micrograph showing a degenerating external hair cell. (From Schuknecht, HF: *Pathology of the Ear.* Harvard University Press, Cambridge, MA, 1974, with permission.)

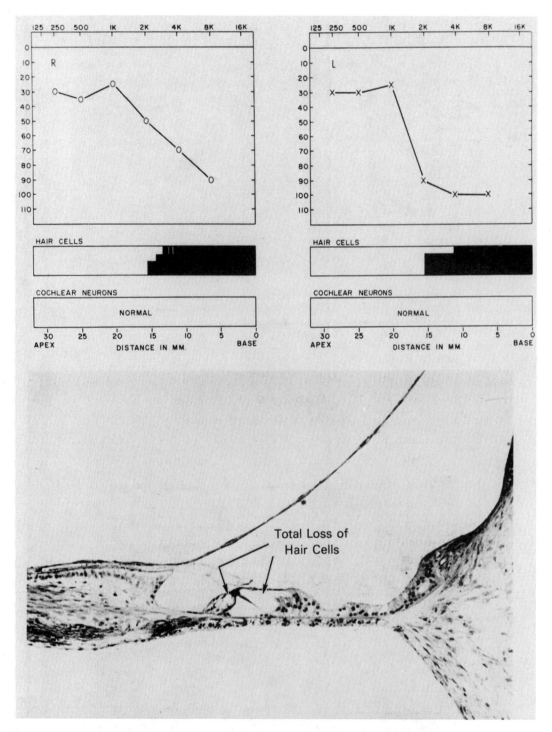

FIGURE 79 Hair cell loss in the cochlea resulting from kanamycin ototoxicity. (*Top*) Correlation between sensorineural hearing loss and hair cell loss (blackened area) along the cochlea; neurons in the ganglion were normal throughout. (*Bottom*) Histopathologic section of the organ of Corti showing total loss of hair cells in the 80-mm region of the cochlea. (From Schuknecht, HF: *Pathology of the Ear.* Harvard University Press, Cambridge, MA, 1974, with permission.)

the crista. Later, type II hair cells are destroyed, but the supporting cells remain unaffected. With the cochleotoxic agents such as kanamycin and amikacin, the outer hair cells in the basal turn of the cochlea are destroyed first, followed by total hair cell loss throughout the cochlea as the dose and duration of treatment are increased.

Patients receiving high-dose salicylate therapy frequently complain of hearing loss, tinnitus, dizziness, loss of balance, and occasionally vertigo.[108] Sensorineural hearing loss involves all frequencies and is associated with recruitment, suggesting a cochlear rather than a nervous system etiology.[109] The tinnitus is high pitched and frequently precedes the onset of hearing loss. Both hearing loss and tinnitus invariably occur when the plasma salicylate level approaches 0.35 mg/mL.[110] Caloric testing often reveals bilaterally depressed responses consistent with bilateral vestibular end organ damage. All symptoms and signs are rapidly reversible after the cessation of salicylate ingestion (usually within 24 hours). As with aminoglycosides, salicylates are highly concentrated in the perilymph, and preliminary evidence suggests that they interfere with enzymatic activity of the hair cells, the cochlear neurons, or both.[111]

The potent diuretics ethacrynic acid and furosemide have clearly documented ototoxic effects.[112] Both drugs produce a rapid-onset sensorineural hearing loss that reverses within hours. Animal studies indicate that these so-called loop-inhibiting diuretics selectively damage the hair cells of the organ of Corti. Combined use of loop-inhibiting diuretics and aminoglycoside antibiotics can lead to a profound permanent hearing loss.

Chemotherapeutic anticancer agents, particularly the alkylating agents, are another group of potent ototoxic drugs.[113] Both the auditory and the vestibular labyrinth are affected, with the main pathological finding being loss of hair cells.

OTOSCLEROSIS

Symptoms	Slowly progressive hearing loss and tinnitus (unilateral or bilateral), family history of similar hearing loss; vertigo, unsteadiness, or both in about one fourth of cases[114]
Signs	Hearing loss, bone conduction greater than air conduction
Laboratory	*Audiometry:* Conductive hearing loss (unilateral or bilateral) (see Fig. 38), restricted tympanogram, abnormal stapedius reflex, BAER usually normal
	ENG: Directional preponderance or vestibular paresis to caloric stimulation in about one half of cases
	CT: Otosclerotic involvement of oval window, round window, or bony labyrinth
Management	*Medical:* Sodium fluoride 40–50 mg/day (give with calcium and vitamin D)[115]
	Amplification: Treatment of choice in many cases
	Surgery: (1) Stapes mobilization (stapediolysis) without removal of any part of the stapes is rarely successful. (2) Subtotal stapedectomy: footplate removed, followed by tissue graft seal of oval window and restoration of part of the stapedial arch. (3) Total stapedectomy: removal of the entire stapedial arch, followed by substitution of a prosthesis linking the incus to the oval window

Otosclerosis, a metabolic disorder that usually has a genetic origin, usually causes conductive hearing loss but may also involve sensorineural hearing loss and vestibular effects.

Otosclerosis is a metabolic disease of the bony labyrinth that usually manifests itself by immobilizing the stapes, thereby producing a conductive hearing loss.[116] A positive family history for otosclerosis is reported in 50% to 70% of cases. The sporadic cases may represent autosomal recessive inheritance or spontaneous mutation or may be nongenetic in origin. Although otosclerosis is primarily a disorder of the auditory system, vestibular symptoms and signs are more common than generally appreciated.

The basic pathological process of otosclerosis is a resorption of normal bone, particularly around blood vessels, and its replacement by cellular, fibrous connective tissue (Fig. 80).[16] With time, immature basophilic bone is produced in the resorption space; after several cycles of resorption and new bone formation, a mature acidophilic bone with laminated matrix is produced.[117] Bilateral involvement is usual but about one fourth of cases are unilateral. Areas of predilection for otosclerotic foci include the oval window region, the round window niche, the anterior wall of the internal auditory canal, and within the stapedial footplate. Although conductive hearing loss is the hallmark of otosclerosis, a combined conductive-sensorineural hearing loss pattern is frequent. The sensorineural component is perhaps caused by foci of otosclerosis next to the spiral ligament of the cochlea, producing atrophy of the

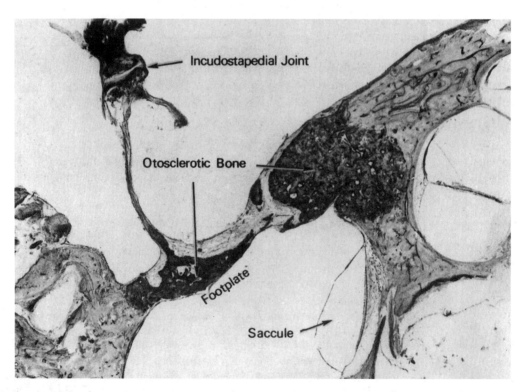

FIGURE 80   Histopathological section showing an otosclerotic lesion involving the bony labyrinth at the anterior margin of the oval window and the entire footplate of the stapes. The patient exhibited a combined conductive-sensorineural hearing loss. (From Schuknecht, HF: *Pathology of the Ear.* Harvard University Press, Cambridge, MA, 1974, with permission.)

spiral ligament. Vestibular symptoms and signs may be caused by mechanical deformation of the labyrinth and vestibular nerve or by biochemical abnormalities of inner ear fluids.[16]

AGING

Presbycusis

Symptoms	Slowly progressive, bilateral hearing loss in the elderly
Signs	Bilateral high-frequency hearing loss
Laboratory	*Audiometry:* Bilateral sensorineural hearing loss; pure tone pattern may be flat, mildly sloping, or severely sloping (see Fig. 39B); occasionally, conductive component also present
Management	Amplification specifically designed for the patient's pattern of hearing loss

The bilateral hearing loss commonly associated with advancing age is called **presbycusis**. Presbycusis is not a distinct entity but rather represents multiple effects of aging on the auditory system.[16] Presbycusis may include conductive and central dysfunction, but the most consistent effect of aging is on the sensory cells and neurons of the cochlea.[118] The typical audiogram of presbycusis is a symmetrical hearing loss gradually sloping downward with increasing frequency. The most consistent pathology associated with presbycusis is a degeneration of sensory cells and nerve fibers at the base of the cochlea.[16]

An audiogram showing a symmetrical hearing loss sloping down with increasing frequency is typical of presbycusis.

Disequilibrium of Aging

Symptoms	Gradually progressive imbalance and unsteadiness when walking; dizziness when standing or walking relieved by sitting or lying down; frequent falls
Signs	Cautious gait with slight widening of the base, shortening of the stride length, and careful slow turns; in later stages, shuffling steps, stooped posture, and lack of associated movements
Laboratory	*ENG:* May show bilateral decreased caloric responses and symmetrical decreased gain to rotational stimulation *MRI:* May show generalized atrophy, enlarged ventricles, subcortical leukoencephalopathy, or midline cerebellar atrophy (Fig. 81)
Management	Physical therapy program aimed at gait and balance training, along with strengthening exercises; scrupulously avoid sedating medications

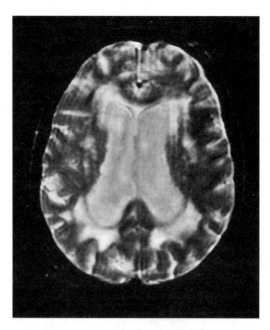

FIGURE 81   MRI (T$_2$-weighted, transverse section) showing subcortical white matter lesions and diffuse cerebral atrophy in a 79-year-old woman with gait unsteadiness and frequent falls.

Minor gait changes are expected with aging, but more severe disorders may be due to neurologic disease, especially multi-infarct syndrome.

The gradual loss of cells in the sensory and motor centers of the brain with aging is usually a very subtle process that parallels similar slight changes in memory and other cognitive functions generally considered the normal aging process. The gait of normal elderly men is characterized by slight anteroflexion of the upper torso with flexion of the arms and knees, diminished arm swing, and shorter step lengths. The gait of older women tends to be narrow based, with a waddling quality. When minor, these changes are not likely to lead to a medical evaluation. A few elderly patients, however, develop a progressive deterioration of gait beginning in the eighth and ninth decades.[119,120] Their steps shorten and their base widens until their gait is reduced to a shuffle. They turn en bloc rather than with a normal pivot, and upon arising they have great difficulty in initiating the first step. Once they begin, their arms are held rigidly at their sides and they exhibit a characteristic stooped posture. Walking in tandem is impossible.

Minor gait abnormalities such as the "cautious gait" have many different causes and so have relatively little diagnostic significance.[121] Such a gait may simply be a compensatory response to any cause of mild imbalance. It can be seen in patients with peripheral neuropathy, after ototoxic drug exposure, or after visual loss or multisensory loss.[122] The more severe gait disorders are associated with neurologic diseases, most commonly due to multi-infarct syndrome.[123] This disorder is most severe in hypertensive patients but also can be seen in normotensive patients over the age of 75.

DEVELOPMENTAL DISORDERS

Maldevelopment of the Inner Ear

Symptoms	Long-standing bilateral hearing loss (onset rarely is delayed to adulthood); subtle balance problems
Signs	Hearing loss plus evidence of associated malformations of the external and/or middle ear, ophthalmic lesions, CNS lesions, skeletal malformations, renal disease, thyroid disease, and miscellaneous congenital defects (In most cases, no other signs are present, however.)
Laboratory	*Audiometry:* Bilateral sensorineural hearing loss with characteristic V-shaped pure tone pattern (see Fig. 39D); BAER often normal unless profound deafness *ENG:* Bilateral decreased caloric responses in approximately one third of cases. *Imaging:* CT identifies a malformed bony labyrinth; MRI identifies malformations of the membranous labyrinth; often no structural abnormalities are found
Management	Amplification where serviceable hearing remains; cochlear implants in selected patients

Although congenital deafness is usually recognized during infancy, congenital vestibular impairment is not because the manifestations are more subtle. Children learn to use other sensory information to compensate for vestibular loss and appear normal on standard developmental tests. Congenital deafness has therefore received extensive study, whereas vestibular loss has been relatively neglected.

Congenital vestibular loss is less likely than deafness to be identified early.

It has been estimated that more than one half of all congenital deafness is inherited, with more than three fourths being inherited in an autosomal recessive fashion.[124] Despite the many recognizable syndromes that have been described, most cases of genetically determined hearing loss are not associated with malformations of other organs or body systems. There have been spectacular advances in the genetic analysis of both syndromic and nonsyndromic congenital hearing loss in the past few years, and one can reasonably expect that most of the abnormal genes will be identified in the next few decades.[125]

The most common cause of acquired congenital malformations of the inner ear is maternal rubella infection during the critical developmental period (the first 9 weeks of gestation for vestibular development and the first 25 weeks for auditory development). Infants born to mothers who acquire rubella in the first trimester of pregnancy may have multiple congenital defects, including cataracts, patent ductus arteriosus, microcephaly, dental defects, and generally impaired growth and development.[126] Hearing loss is more common than is vestibular loss, apparently because of the longer critical developmental period. Less often, the infant's fully developed inner ear may be damaged by maternal rubella infection in the last two trimesters.[127] Other important causes of acquired congenital inner ear defects include maternal drug or toxin ingestion, hyperbilirubinemia, anoxia associated with difficult birth, and cretinism.[16]

Chiari Malformation

Symptoms   Oscillopsia and gait unsteadiness

Signs   Spontaneous nystagmus (typically downbeat), lower cranial nerve palsies, gait
                    and extremity ataxia

Laboratory   *ENG:* Downbeat nystagmus increases on lateral gaze, no change with loss of
                    fixation; impaired smooth pursuit and optokinetic nystagmus, impaired fixation
                    suppression of vestibular nystagmus
                    MRI: Herniation of cerebellar tonsils into foramen magnum best seen on thin
                    sagittal sections (Fig. 82)

Management   Suboccipital decompression of foramen magnum region[128]

A Chiari type I malformation may first manifest itself in adulthood with gait unsteadiness and oscillopsia.

Most frequently the Chiari malformation manifests itself in the first few months of life and is associated with hydrocephalus and other nervous system malformations (type II malformation). Less frequent but more important to the neurotologist are those cases in which the onset of symptoms and signs is delayed until adulthood (type I malformation). These cases often present with subtle neurologic symptoms and signs and are usually unassociated with other developmental defects. The most common neurotological symptom is a slowly progressive unsteadiness of gait that the pa-

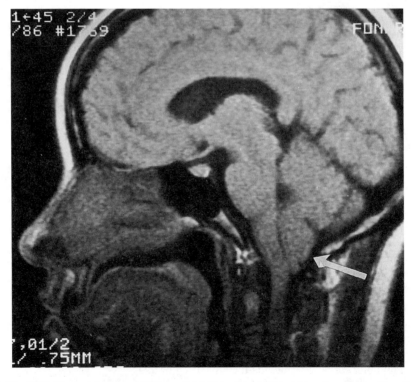

FIGURE 82 MRI (T$_1$-weighted, sagittal section) showing a Chiari type I malformation. Arrow points to the cerebellar tonsils herniating into the foramen magnum.

tient frequently describes as dizziness. Vertigo and hearing loss occur in about 10% of patients.[129] Oscillopsia is nearly always present, owing to the spontaneous vertical downbeat nystagmus. Dysphagia, hoarseness, and dysarthria result from stretching of the lower cranial nerves, and obstructive hydrocephalus can result from occlusion of the basilar cisterns.[130]

MULTIPLE SCLEROSIS

Symptoms	Monocular visual loss, vertigo, double vision, weakness, numbness, and ataxia
Signs	Involvement of pyramidal tracts (hyperreflexia, extensor plantar responses), cerebellum (intention tremor, ataxia, slurred speech), sensory tracts (impaired vibratory and position sense), and visual pathways (decreased visual acuity and pallor of the optic disc); many varieties of pathological nystagmus, most commonly dissociated nystagmus on lateral gaze and acquired spontaneous pendular nystagmus
Laboratory	*Audiometry:* BAER can detect subclinical lesions
	ENG: May show abnormalities of saccades, smooth pursuit, and visuovestibular interaction
	CSF: Elevated γ-globulin levels with oligoclonal bands
	MRI: Usually shows characteristic T_2 intense lesions in the subcortical white matter (Fig. 83)
Management	Steroids can accelerate remissions after exacerbations, and interferon-β decreases the number of exacerbations, but so far no treatment clearly alters the natural history of the disease

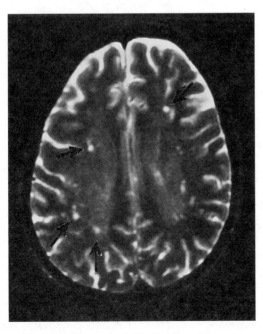

FIGURE 83 MRI (T_2-weighted, transverse section) demonstrating deep white matter lesions (arrows) in a patient with multiple sclerosis.

Multiple sclerosis (MS) is a demyelinating disease of the central nervous system of unknown cause, with onset usually in the third or fourth decades of life.[131] The key to the diagnosis is the finding of disseminated signs of CNS dysfunction manifested in an alternating remitting and exacerbating course. Although many symptoms occur with MS, certain ones deserve emphasis because of their consistent appearance. Blurring or loss of vision caused by demyelination of the optic nerve (retrobulbar neuritis) is the initial symptom in about 20% of patients. Vertigo is the initial symptom in about 5% of patients and is reported at some time during the disease in as many as 50%.[132] Hearing loss occurs in about 10% of patients.[133]

The demyelination in MS is confined to CNS myelin, the myelin produced by oligodendrogliocytes. Because both peripheral and cranial nerves contain CNS myelin at their root entry zones, a demyelinating plaque involving the root entry zone may produce signs of peripheral nerve dysfunction. Plaques involving the vestibular and auditory nerve root entry zones can explain the frequent findings of unilateral caloric hypoexcitability and unilateral hearing loss in patients with MS.

References

1. Ingarsson L, Lundgren K, and Stenstrom C: Occurrence of acute otitis media in children: Cohort studies in an urban population. Ann Otol Rhinol Laryngol 149 (Suppl):1, 1990.
2. Henderson FW, Collier AM, Sanyal MA, et al.: A longitudinal study of respiratory viruses and bacteria in the etiology of acute otitis media with effusion. N Engl J Med 396:1377, 1982.
3. Sarkkinen H, Ruuskaneno L, Meurman O, et al.: Identification of respiratory virus antigens in the middle ear fluids of children with acute otitis media. J Infect Dis 151:444, 1985.
4. McCabe W: The correlation of in vitro tests with the outcome of automicrobial therapy for otitis media. Pediatr Ann 13:365, 1984.
5. Smyth GDL: Tympanomastoid disease. In Gibb AL, and Smith MFW (eds): Otology (Butterworths International Reviews). Butterworths, London, 1982.
6. Paparella M, Oda M, Hiraide F, and Brady D: Pathology of sensorineural hearing loss in otitis media. Ann Otol Rhinol Laryngol 81:632, 1972.
7. Bhaya MH, Schachern PA, Morizono T, and Paparella MM: Pathogenesis of tympanosclerosis. Otolaryngol Head Neck Surg 109:413, 1993.
8. Chole RA: Osteoclasts in chronic otitis media, cholesteatoma and otosclerosis. Ann Otol Rhinol Laryngol 97:661, 1988.
9. Jahn AF, and Hawke M: Infections of the external ear. In Cummings CW, et al. (eds): Otolaryngology—Head and Neck Surgery, ed 2. C.V. Mosby, St. Louis, 1993.
10. Hickey SA, Ford GR, Eykyn SJ, et al.: Treating malignant external otitis with ciprofloxacin. BMJ 299:550, 1989.
11. McShane D, Chapnik JS, Noyek AM, and Vellend H: Malignant external otitis. J Otolaryngol 15:2, 1986.
12. Neely JG: Complications of temporal bone infection. In Cummings CW, et al. (eds): Otolaryngology—Head and Neck Surgery, ed 2. C.V. Mosby, St. Louis, 1993.
13. Gower D, and McGuirt WF: Intracranial complications of acute and chronic infectious ear disease: A problem still with us. Laryngoscope 93:1028, 1983.
14. Schwaber MK, Pensak ML, and Bartels JL: The early signs and symptoms of neurotologic complications of chronic suppurative otitis media. Laryngoscope 99:373, 1989.
15. Paparella MM, Goycoolea MV, and Meyerhoff WL: Inner ear pathology and otitis media: A review. Ann Otol Rhinol Laryngol 89:249, 1980.

16. Schuknecht HF: Pathology of the Ear, ed 2. Lea & Febiger, Philadelphia, 1993.
17. Ariyasu L, Byl FM, Sprague MS, and Adour KK: The beneficial effect of methylprednisone in acute vestibular vertigo. Arch Otolaryngol Head Neck Surg 116:700, 1990.
18. Schuknecht HF: Neurolabyrinthitis. Viral infections of the peripheral auditory and vestibular systems. In Nomura Y (ed): Hearing Loss and Dizziness. Igaku-Shoin, Tokyo, 1985.
19. Wilson WR, Veltri RW, Laird N, and Sprinkle PM: Viral and epidemiologic studies of idiopathic sudden hearing loss. Otolaryngol Head Neck Surg 91:653, 1983.
20. Böhmer A: Acute unilateral peripheral vestibulopathy. In Baloh RW, and Halmagyi GM (eds): Disorders of the Vestibular System. Oxford University Press, New York, 1996.
21. Baloh RW, Lopez I, Ishiyama A, et al.: Vestibular neuritis: Clinical-pathologic correlation. Otolaryngol Head Neck Surg 114:586, 1996.
22. Nomura Y, Kurata T, and Saito K: Sudden deafness: Human temporal bones studies and an animal model. In Nomura Y (ed): Hearing Loss and Dizziness. Igaku-Shoin, Tokyo, 1985.
23. Portmann M, Dauman R, and Aran JM: Audiometric and electrophysiological correlations in sudden deafness. Acta Otolaryngol 99:363, 1985.
24. Rahko T, and Karma P: New clinical finding in vestibular neuritis: High frequency audiometry hearing loss in the affected ear. Laryngoscope 96:198, 1986.
25. Wilson WR, Laird N, and Kavesh DA: Electronystagmographic findings in idiopathic sudden hearing loss. Am J Otolaryngol 3:279, 1982.
26. Dickens JRE, Smith JT, and Grotlam SS: Herpes zoster oticus: Treatment with intravenous acyclovir. Laryngoscope 98:776, 1988.
27. Robillard RB, Hilsinger RL, and Adour KK: Ramsay Hunt facial paralysis: Clinical analysis of 185 patients. Otolaryngol Head Neck Surg 95:292, 1986.
28. Zajtchuk J, Matz G, and Lindsay J: Temporal bone pathology in herpes oticus. Ann Otol Rhinol Laryngol 81:331, 1972.
29. Hughes GB, and Rutherford I: Predictive value of serologic tests for syphilis in otology. Ann Otol Rhinol Laryngol 95:250, 1986.
30. Morrison AW: Late syphilis. In Morrison AW (ed): Management of Sensorineural Deafness. Butterworths, Boston, 1975.
31. Steckelberg JM, and McDonald TJ: Otologic involvement in late syphilis. Laryngoscope 94:753, 1984.
32. Polus K: The problem of vascular deafness. Laryngoscope 82:24, 1972.
33. Baloh RW, and Honrubia V: Clinical Neurophysiology of the Vestibular System, ed 2. F.A. Davis, Philadelphia, 1990.
34. Andrews J, Hoover LA, Lee RS, and Honrubia V: Vertigo in the hyperviscosity syndrome. Otolaryngol Head Neck Surg 98:144, 1988.
35. Linsay JR, and Hemenway WG: Postural vertigo due to unilateral sudden partial loss of vestibular function. Ann Otol Rhinol Laryngol 65:692, 1956.
36. Paparella M, Berlinger NT, Oda M, and el-Fiky F: Otological manifestations of leukemia. Laryngoscope 83:1510, 1973.
37. Fisher CM: Vertigo in cerebrovascular disease. Arch Otolaryngol 85:855, 1967.
38. Grad A, and Baloh RW: Vertigo of vascular origin: Clinical and ENG features of 84 cases. Arch Neurol 46:281, 1989.
39. Fife TD, Baloh RW, and Duckwiler GR: Isolated dizziness in vertebrobasilar insufficiency. Clinical features, angiography, and follow-up. J Stroke Cerebrovasc Dis 4:4, 1994.
40. Caplan LR: Vertebrobasilar disease. In Barnett HJM, et al. (eds): Stroke: Pathophysiology, Diagnosis and Management. Churchill Livingstone, New York, 1986.
41. Bogousslavsky J, Fox AJ, Barnett HJM, et al.: Clinicotopographic correlation of small vertebrobasilar infarct using magnetic resonance imaging. Stroke 17:929, 1986.
42. Fisher CM, Karnes WE, and Kubik CS: Lateral medullary infarction—the pattern of vascular occlusion. J Neuropathol Exp Neurol 20:323, 1961.
43. Bjerner K, and Silfverskiold BP: Lateropulsion an imbalance in Wallenberg's syndrome. Acta Neurol Scand 44:91, 1968.
44. Kommerell G, and Hoyt WF: Lateropulsion of saccadic eye movements. Electrooculographic studies in a patient with Wallenberg's syndrome. Arch Neurol 28:313, 1973.

45. Oas J, and Baloh RW: Vertigo and the anterior inferior cerebellar artery syndrome. Neurology 42:2274, 1992.
46. Amarenco P, and Hauw J-J: Cerebellar infarction in the territory of the anterior and inferior cerebellar artery: A clinico-pathological study of 20 cases. Brain 113:139, 1990.
47. Barth A, Bogousslavsky J, and Regli F: The clinical and topographic spectrum of cerebellar infarcts: A clinical-magnetic resonance imaging correlation study. Ann Neurol 33:451, 1993.
48. Caplan LR: Brain embolism, revisited. Neurology 43:1281, 1993.
49. Amarenco P, and Hauw J-J: Cerebellar infarction in the territory of the superior cerebellar artery: A clinico-pathological study of 33 cases. Neurology 40:1383, 1990.
50. Baloh RW: Vestibular disorders due to cerebrovascular disease. In Baloh RW, and Halmagyi GM (eds): Disorders of the Vestibular System. Oxford University Press, New York, 1996.
51. Ott KH, Kase CS, Ojemann RG, and Mohr JP: Cerebellar hemorrhage: Diagnosis and treatment. Arch Neurol 31:160, 1974.
52. Brennen RW, and Bergland RM: Acute cerebellar hemorrhage. Analysis of clinical findings and outcome in 12 cases. Neurology 27:527, 1977.
53. Baloh RW: Benign positional vertigo. In Baloh RW, and Halmagyi GM (eds): Disorders of the Vestibular System. Oxford University Press, New York, 1996.
54. Baloh RW, Honrubia V, and Jacobson K: Benign positional vertigo. Clinical and oculographic features in 240 cases. Neurology 37:371, 1987.
55. Cohen B, Suzuki J, and Bender MB: Eye movements from semicircular canal nerve stimulation in the cat. Ann Otol Rhinol Laryngol 73:153, 1964.
56. Hall SF, Ruby SRF, and McClure JA: The mechanics of benign paroxysmal vertigo. J Otolaryngol 8:151, 1979.
57. Epley JM: The canalith repositioning procedure: For treatment of benign paroxysmal positional vertigo. Otolaryngol Head Neck Surg 107:399, 1992.
58. Brandt T, and Steddin S: Current view of the mechanism of benign paroxysmal positional vertigo: Cupulolithiasis or canalithiasis? J Vestib Res 3:373, 1993.
59. Gacek RR: Singular neurectomy update II. Review of 102 cases. Laryngoscope 101:855, 1991.
60. Parnes LS, and McClure JA: Free floating endolymphatic particles: A new operative finding during posterior semicircular canal occlusion. Laryngoscope 102:988, 1992.
61. McClure JA: Horizontal canal BPV. J Otolaryngol 14:30, 1985.
62. Pagnini P, Nute D, and Vannucchi P: Benign paroxysmal vertigo of the horizontal canal. ORL J Otorhinolaryngol Relat Spec 51:161, 1989.
63. Baloh RW, Jacobson K, and Honrubia V: Horizontal canal variant of benign positional vertigo. Neurology 43:2542, 1993.
64. McClure JA, and Parnes LS: A cure for benign positional vertigo. In Baloh RW (ed): Bailliere's Clinical Neurology: Neurotology. Bailliere Tindall, London, 1994.
65. Santos PM, Hall RA, Snyder JM, et al.: Diuretic and diet effect on Ménière's disease evaluated by the 1989 Committee on Hearing and Equilibrium guidelines. Otolaryngol Head Neck Surg 109:680, 1993.
66. Bergenius J, and Odkvist LM: Transtympanic aminoglycoside treatment of Ménière's disease. In Baloh RW, and Halmagyi GM (eds): Disorders of the Vestibular System. Oxford University Press, New York, 1996.
67. Brackmann DE: Surgical procedures: Endolymphatic shunt, vestibular nerve section, and labyrinthectomy. In Baloh RW, and Halmagyi GM (eds): Disorders of the Vestibular System. Oxford University Press, New York, 1996.
68. Andrews JC, and Honrubia V: Ménière's disease. In Baloh RW, and Halmagyi GM (eds): Disorders of the Vestibular System. Oxford University Press, New York, 1996.
69. Rassekh CH, and Harker LA: The prevalence of migraine in Ménière's disease. Laryngoscope 102:135, 1992.
70. Schuknecht HF: Delayed endolymphatic hydrops. Ann Otol Rhinol Laryngol 87:743, 1978.
71. Baloh RW, Jacobson K, and Winder T: Drop attacks with Ménière's disease. Ann Neurol 28:384, 1990.
72. Moscicki RA: Immune mediated inner ear disorders. In Baloh RW (ed): Neurotology. Bailliere Tindall, London, 1994.
73. Bloch DB, San Martin JE, Rauch SD, et al.: Serum antibodies to heat

shock protein 70 in sensorineural hearing loss. Arch Otolaryngol Head Neck Surg 121:1167, 1995.

74. Harris JP: Immunologic mechanisms in disorders of the inner ear. In Cummings CW, et al. (eds): Otolaryngology—Head and Neck Surgery, ed 2. C.V. Mosby, St. Louis, 1993.

75. Harris JP, and O'Driscoll K: Autoimmune inner ear disease. In Baloh RW, and Halmagyi GM (eds): Disorders of the Vestibular System. Oxford University Press, New York, 1996.

76. Kayan A, and Hood JD: Neuro-otological manifestations of migraine. Brain 107:1123, 1984.

77. Harker LA, and Rassek HC: Episodic vertigo in basilar migraine. Otolaryngol Head Neck Surg 96:239, 1987.

78. Viirre E, and Baloh RW: Migraine as a cause of sudden hearing loss. Headache 36:24, 1996.

79. Olesen J: Headache Classification Committee of the International Headache Society: Classification and diagnostic criteria for headache disorders, cranial neuralgias and facial pain. Cephalalgia 8 (Suppl 7):1, 1988.

80. Atkinson M: Ménière's syndrome and migraine: Observations on a causal relationship. Ann Intern Med 18:797, 1943.

81. Ophoff RA, Terwindt GM, Vergouwe MN, et al: Familial hemiplegic migraine and episodic ataxia type-2 are caused by mutations in the Ca^{++} channel gene CACNL1A4. Cell 87:543, 1996.

82. Haan J, Terwindt GM, Ophoff RA, et al.: Is familial hemiplegic migraine a hereditary form of basilar migraine? Cephalalgia 15:477, 1995.

83. Thawley SE, and Panje WR (eds): Comprehensive Management of Head and Neck Tumors. W.B. Saunders, Philadelphia, 1987.

84. Stell PM, and McCormick MS: Carcinoma of the external auditory meatus and middle ear. Prognostic factors and a suggested staging system. J Laryngol Otol 99:847, 1985.

85. Brown JS: Glomus jugulare tumors revisited: A ten-year statistical follow-up of 231 cases. Laryngoscope 95:284, 1985.

86. Mattox DE: Vestibular schwannomas. Otolaryngol Clin North Am 20:149, 1987.

87. Kim HN, and Jenkins HA: Vestibular schwannomas and other cerebellopontine angle tumors. In Baloh RW, and Halmagyi GM (eds): Disorders of the Vestibular System. Oxford University Press, New York, 1996.

88. Brackmann DE, and Bartels LJ: Rare tumors of the cerebellopontine angle. Otolaryngol Head Neck Surg 88:555, 1980.

89. Gherini SG, Brackmann DE, Lo WW, and Solti-Bohman LG: Cholesterol granuloma of the petrous apex. Laryngoscope 95:6, 1985.

90. Bradac GB, Schorner W, Bevder A, and Felix R: MRI (NMR) in the diagnosis of brain tumors. Neuroradiology 27:208, 1985.

91. Hirose G, and Halmagyi GM: Brain tumors and balance disorders. In Baloh RW, and Halmagyi GM (eds): Disorders of the Vestibular System. Oxford University Press, New York, 1996.

92. Poereskin L, and Treip C: Adult medulloblastoma. J Neurol Neurosurg Psychiatry 49:39, 1986.

93. Grand W: Positional nystagmus: An early sign of medulloblastoma. Neurology 21:1157, 1971.

94. Gregorius FK, Crandall PH, and Baloh RW: Positional vertigo in cerebellar astrocytoma: Report of two cases. Surg Neurol 6:283, 1976.

95. Jaffe BF: Vertigo following air travel. N Engl J Med 301:1385, 1979.

96. Gacek RR: Perilymphatic fistula. In Cummings CW, et al. (eds): Otolaryngology—Head and Neck Surgery, ed 2. C.V. Mosby, St. Louis, 1993.

97. Goodhill V: Leaking labyrinth lesions, deafness, tinnitus, and dizziness. Ann Otol Rhinol Laryngol 90:99, 1981.

98. Schuknecht HF: Cochleosacculotomy for Ménière's disease: Theory, techniques and results. Laryngoscope 92:853, 1982.

99. Davey LM: Labyrinthine trauma in head injury. Conn Med 29:250, 1965.

100. Igarashi M, Schuknecht H, and Myers E: Cochlear pathology in humans with stimulation deafness. J Laryngol 78:1125, 1964.

101. Schuknecht H, Neff W, and Perlman H: An experimental study of auditory damage following blows to the head. Ann Otol Rhinol Laryngol 60:273, 1951.

102. Cooper JC, and Owen JH: Audiologic profile of noise-induced hearing loss. Arch Otolaryngol 102:148, 1976.

103. Fee WE: Aminoglycoside ototoxicity in the human. Laryngoscope 24 (Suppl):1, 1980.

104. Smith CR, Lipsky JJ, Laskin OL, et al.: Double blind comparison of the

nephrotoxicity and auditory toxicity of gentamicin and tobramycin. N Engl J Med 302:1106, 1980.

105. Rybak LP, and Matz GJ: Effects of toxic agents. In Cummings CW, et al. (eds): Otolaryngology—Head and Neck Surgery, ed 2. C.V. Mosby, St. Louis, 1993.

106. Lerner SA, and Matz GJ: Aminoglycoside ototoxicity. Am J Otolaryngol 1:169, 1980.

107. Hutchin T, and Cortopassi TG: Proposed molecular and cellular mechanism for aminoglycoside ototoxicity. Antimicrob Agents Chemother 38:2517, 1994.

108. Myers E, Bernstein J, and Fostiropolous G: Salicylate ototoxicity. A clinical study. N Engl J Med 273:587, 1965.

109. McCabe P, and Dey F: The effect of aspirin upon auditory sensitivity. Ann Otol Rhinol Laryngol 74:312, 1965.

110. Day RO, Graham G, Bieri D, et al.: Concentration-response relationships for salicylate induced ototoxicity in normal volunteers. Br J Clin Pharmacol 28:695, 1989.

111. Silverstein H, Berstein J, and Davies D: Salicylate ototoxicity. A biochemical and electrophysiological study. Ann Otol Rhinol Laryngol 76:118, 1967.

112. Mathog RH, Thomas WG, and Hudson WR: Ototoxicity of new and potent diuretics. Arch Otolaryngol 92:7, 1970.

113. Hess K: Vestibulotoxic drugs and other causes of acquired bilateral peripheral vestibulopathy. In Baloh RW, and Halmagyi GM (eds): Disorders of the Vestibular System. Oxford University Press, New York, 1996.

114. Cody DTR, and Baker HL: Otosclerosis: Vestibular symptoms and sensorineural hearing loss. Ann Otol Rhinol Laryngol 87:778, 1978.

115. Snow JB Jr: Current status of fluoride therapy for otosclerosis. Am J Otol 6:56, 1985.

116. Donaldson JA, and Snyder JM: Otosclerosis. In Cummings CW, et al. (eds): Otolaryngology—Head and Neck Surgery, ed 2. C.V. Mosby, St. Louis, 1993.

117. Lim DJ: Pathogenesis and pathology of otosclerosis: A review. In Nomura Y (ed): Hearing Loss and Dizziness. Igaku-Shoin, Tokyo, 1985.

118. Johnson L, and Hawkins J: Sensory and neural degeneration with aging, as seen in microdissections of the human inner ear. Ann Otol Rhinol Laryngol 81:179, 1972.

119. Bloem BR, Haan J, Lagaay AM, et al.: Investigation of gait in elderly subjects over 88 years of age. J Geriatr Psychiatry Neurol 5:78, 1992.

120. Elble RJ, Hughes L, and Higgins C: The syndrome of senile gait. J Neurol 239:71, 1992.

121. Nutt J, Marsden CD, and Thompson PD: Human walking and higher-level gait disorders, particularly in the elderly. Neurology 43:268, 1993.

122. Fife TD, and Baloh RW: Disequilibrium of unknown cause in older people. Ann Neurol 34:674, 1993.

123. Thompson PD, and Marsden CD: Gait disorder of subcortical arteriosclerotic encephalopathy: Binswanger's disease. Mov Disord 2:1, 1987.

124. Brookhauser PE: Sensorineural hearing loss in children. In Cummings CW, et al. (eds): Otolaryngology—Head and Neck Surgery, ed 2. C.V. Mosby, St. Louis, 1993.

125. Baloh RW: Vestibular and auditory disorders. Curr Opin Neurol 9:32, 1996.

126. Barr B, and Lundstrom R: Deafness following maternal rubella. Acta Otolaryngol 53:413, 1961.

127. Monif G, Hardy J, and Sever J: Studies in congenital rubella, Baltimore 1964–1965. I. Epidemiologic and virologic. Bull Johns Hopkins Hosp 118:85, 1966.

128. Spooner JW, and Baloh RW: Arnold-Chiari malformation: Improvement in eye movements after surgical treatment. Brain 104:51, 1981.

129. Saez RJ, Onofrio BM, and Yanagihara T: Experience with Arnold-Chiari formation: 1960 to 1970. J Neurosurg 45:416, 1975.

130. Paul KS, Lye RH, Strang FA, and Dutton J: Arnold-Chiari malformation: Review of 71 cases. J Neurosurg 58:183, 1983.

131. McAlpine D, Lumsden CE, and Acheson ED: Multiple Sclerosis: A Reappraisal. Churchill Livingstone, Edinburgh and London, 1972.

132. Grenman R: Involvement of the audiovestibular system in multiple sclerosis: An otoneurologic and audiologic study. Acta Otolaryngol Suppl 420:9, 1985.

133. Noffsinger D, Olsen WO, Carhart R, et al.: Auditory and vestibular aberrations in multiple sclerosis. Acta Otolaryngol Suppl 303:7, 1972.

11

Symptomatic Treatment of Vertigo

The best therapy for vertigo is to eliminate it by treating the underlying illness (see Chapter 10). When the illness is not readily treatable, however, when treatment must be continued for a long period before improvement occurs, or when vertigo is prolonged and severe, symptomatic therapy is needed.

The ideal symptomatic treatment of vertigo should suppress the sensation of vertigo, help restore normal balance, and prevent vomiting. Side effects should be minimal, and treatment should not impede the normal process of recovery from vestibular illness. No medication is now available that meets all these ideals. In the absence of an ideal drug, the choice of therapy should take into account the patient's underlying disease, the expected course of the illness, and the patient's need for mobility during recovery.

If the illness underlying a patient's vertigo cannot readily be eliminated, then other therapy is needed to suppress the disabling symptoms.

DRUG TREATMENT

Two types of drugs are used in the symptomatic treatment of vertigo. **Vestibular suppressants** treat a broad variety of symptoms associated with vestibular illness, usually controlling both the sensation of vertigo and any associated nausea. **Antiemetics** are more selective in action; they are used primarily to control nausea and vomiting and are often used in combination with antivertiginous drugs.

Table 20 **Vestibular Suppressants**

Chemical Name	Brand Name	Form and Dosage	Efficacy		Precautions
			Sedative	Antiemetic	
Antihistamines					
Diphenhydramine	Benadryl (OTC)	PO: 25–50 mg q 4–6 h IM/IV: 10–50 mg q.i.d.	+	+	Asthma, glaucoma, prostate enlargement
Dimenhydrinate	Dramamine (OTC)	PO: 50 mg q 4–6 h	+	+	Same
Cyclizine	Marezine (OTC)	PO: 50 mg q 4–6 h	+	+	Same
Meclizine	Antivert Bonine (OTC)	PO: 25–50 mg qd–q.i.d.	±	+	Same
Promethazine	Phenergan	PO: 25 mg q 6 h Supp: 50 mg q 12 h IM: 25 mg q 4–6 h	++	++	Same; history of seizures
Benzodiazepines					
Diazepam	Valium	PO: 2/5/10 mg b.i.d.–q.i.d. Slow IV: 5–10 mg q 4 h	+++	+	Untreated glaucoma, history of drug addiction, pregnancy
Lorazepam	Ativan	PO: 1–2 mg t.i.d. IM/slow IV: 2 mg	+++	+	Same
Clonazepam	Klonopin	PO: 0.5 mg t.i.d.	+++	+	Same
Butyrophenone					
Droperidol	Inapsine	IM/slow IV: 2.5–5 mg q 12 h	+++	++	Liver or kidney disease

OTC = available over the counter.

Vestibular Suppressant Drugs

Mechanisms of Action

The major classes of vestibular suppressants include antihistamines, benzodiazepines, and anticholinergics, although a variety of other drugs also have been used (Table 20).[1] Abundant experimental evidence now demonstrates the efficacy of these medications in the treatment of vertigo. Although the exact mechanism of action of many of these drugs is unclear, most appear to act at the level of the neurotransmitters involved in propagation of impulses from primary to secondary vestibular neurons and in maintainence of tone in the vestibular nuclei. Acetylcholine is an important excitatory neurotransmitter in the vestibular system; muscarinic receptors in the vestibular nuclei are the presumed site of action for anticholinergic-type vestibular suppressants. A major histaminergic system projects to the vestibular nuclei and brain stem autonomic centers, but most antihistamines used to treat vertigo also have an anticholinergic action.[2] The benzodiazepines used to treat vertigo are agonists of gamma-aminobutyric acid (GABA), which is the primary inhibitory neurotransmitter for vestibular neurons.[3]

Most vestibular suppressant drugs effective against vertigo appear to work by acting on the relevant neurotransmitters.

Choice of Vestibular Suppressants

Drugs used in the symptomatic treatment of vertigo can be used either acutely to treat a discrete attack or chronically as prophylaxis against future attacks. To decrease the risk of unacceptable side effects, the choice of drug and method of administration must be determined according to the underlying vestibular illness.

Acute, severe attacks of vertigo accompanied by nausea and vomiting tend to be the most distressing form of vestibular illness. Acute treatment is useful only for those attacks that last long enough for the drug to reach an effective blood level before the attack ends. This limits acute therapy to attacks lasting at least 30 minutes. Since maximal vestibular suppression may not be reached for 2 or more hours after dosing,[4] treatment is most useful for attacks that last several hours. Extremely brief vertigo spells, such as those caused by benign positional vertigo (BPV), cannot be controlled by ingestion of a suppressant at the time the attack begins.

Chronic prophylactic treatment with vestibular suppressants should be used when moderate to severe attacks recur on a frequent basis. During long-term therapy, one must balance the need to control vertigo against the need for the patient to maintain full mobility and function. One of the milder suppressants can be used on a daily basis to "take the edge off" the attacks, adding acute antiemetic treatment if spells are very prolonged or are associated with vomiting. In general, the stronger suppressants are more sedating and should be reserved for acute treatment (Table 21). Some persons experience vestibular symptoms on an almost continuous daily basis. It is difficult to manage these patients with symptomatic treatment alone; efforts should be directed at diagnosis and treatment of the underlying medical condition. Vestibular suppressant medications are not indicated to treat chronic dizziness of nonvestibular origin.

Acute treatment is most useful for attacks that last several hours.

The choice of drugs for chronic prophylactic treatment must consider side effects such as sedation.

Table 21 Indications for Use of Common Vestibular Suppressants

	Acute Peripheral Vertigo	Chronic Recurrent Peripheral Vertigo	Central Vertigo	Prevent Motion Sickness
Less Sedating				
Scopolamine hydrobromide		+		+
Meclizine		+		+
Cyclizine		+		+
Dimenhydrinate		+		+
Diphenhydramine		+		+
More Sedating				
Promethazine	+			+
Diazepam	+		+	
Lorazepam	+		+	
Droperidol	+		+	

Sudden, permanent vestibular injury requires careful management. Because the injury is permanent, compensation must occur before recovery will be complete. All vestibular suppressants impair the process of compensation. Patients are often extremely vertiginous and nauseated for the first few days, and it is appropriate to use stronger vestibular suppressants or antiemetics at this time. As soon as vomiting ceases, however, all suppressants should be withdrawn in order to stimulate normal compensation. A course of vestibular rehabilitation (discussed later) is the appropriate therapy in these cases.

> *Vestibular suppressants impair compensation and must not be used for more than a few days after a sudden, permanent vestibular injury.*

Antiemetic Drugs

Mechanisms of Action

Antiemetic drugs are directed specifically against the areas of the nervous system controlling vomiting (Fig. 84). This system of neurons contains both central components (loosely identified as the **emetic center**) and peripheral components in the GI tract itself. Dopamine, histamine, acetylcholine, and serotonin are all neurotransmitters believed to act at these sites to produce vomiting. Most of the vestibular suppressants have anticholinergic or antihistaminic qualities, giving them antiemetic properties in addition to their effect on vertigo.

The emetic center is not a discrete, localized area in the brain. The final processes involved in emesis seem to be coordinated in the reticular formation of the brain stem, but input is received from numerous areas of the brain stem and cortex. The chemoreceptor trigger zone, located in the area postrema, is a major relay in triggering emesis.[2] Many antiemetics act by suppressing activity in the reticular formation or area postrema. Others suppress major

> *General antiemetics may relieve vomiting associated with vertigo by blocking the brain stem emetic center.*

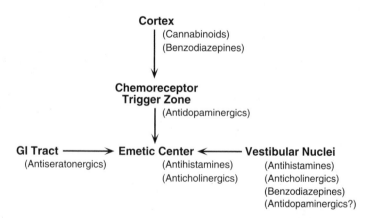

Cortex
(Cannabinoids)
(Benzodiazepines)

↓

Chemoreceptor Trigger Zone
(Antidopaminergics)

↓

GI Tract → **Emetic Center** ← **Vestibular Nuclei**
(Antiseratonergics) (Antihistamines) (Antihistamines)
                     (Anticholinergics) (Anticholinergics)
                                          (Benzodiazepines)
                                          (Antidopaminergics?)

FIGURE 84 Schematic drawing of the major inputs to the emetic center and probable site of action of different classes of drugs. (Adapted from Baloh, RW: Antiemetic and antivertiginous drugs. In Rowland, LP and Klein, DF: *Current Neurologic Drugs.* Current Medicine, Philadelphia, 1996, p. 172, with permission.)

centers feeding into the emesis center or affect peripheral input from the GI tract. Although the exact pathways mediating vestibularly induced vomiting are not known, people who are particularly susceptible to such stimuli also demonstrate increased responses to other emetic center stimuli.[5] This provides a rationale for the use of general antiemetics in vertigo associated with nausea.

Choice of Antiemetics

When nausea and vomiting are prominent, a mild vestibular suppressant can be combined with an antiemetic to control symptoms (Table 22). These medications all have central dopamine antagonist properties and are believed to prevent emesis by inhibition at the chemoreceptor trigger zone (see Fig. 84).

The central antidopaminergic effects of these medications occasionally give rise to serious side effects in patients, particularly in young persons. Although the incidence is less than 1% to 2% in older adults, in young adults and children the incidence can be as high as 25%.[6,7] Since these reactions frequently develop during the first few days of treatment, the treating physician should be prepared to recognize and treat them. The major reactions can be categorized symptomatically as parkinsonism, akathisia, dystonia, and dyskinesia. The latter can be acute and reversible or subacute (tardive) and prolonged or permanent. An individual patient can display characteristics of more than one form.[8]

> *Physicians should watch out for serious side effects when prescribing medications with central dopaminergic effects, especially for young people.*

Selecting the Right Drug

As a general rule, the usefulness of the different symptomatic treatments of vertigo has been determined by empirical observa-

---

Table 22 **Primary Antiemetics**

	Prochlorperazine	Chlorpromazine	Metoclopramide
Brand Name	Compazine	Thorazine	Reglan, Octamide, Maxolon
Class	Phenothiazine	Phenothiazine	Benzamide
Form and Dosage	PO: 5–10 mg q 6 h	PO: 10–25 mg q 6 h	PO: 5–10 mg q.i.d.
	Supp: 25 mg q 12 h	Supp: 50–100 mg q 6–8 h	IM: 10 mg q 4–6 h
	IM: 5–10 mg q 6 h	IM: 25 mg q 3–4 h	IV: 10 mg q 4–6 h
	IV: 2.5–10 mg slow		
Sedative Efficacy	+	+++	+
Antiemetic Efficacy	+++	++	+++
*Extrapyramidal Side Effects**	++	+++	+
Precautions	Liver disease; additive with other CNS depressants; do not use with benzamides	Same as for prochlorperazine	Liver or renal disease; seizures, bowel obstruction, pheochromocytoma; do not use with phenothiazines or in children

*Dystonia, dyskinesia, akathisia, parkinsonism.

tion. The strategy for deciding which drug or combination of drugs to use is based on the known effects of each drug (see Tables 20 and 22) and on the severity and time course of symptoms. In patients with acute severe vertigo, sedation is desirable and drugs such as promethazine and diazepam are particularly useful. If nausea and vomiting are severe, the antiemetics prochlorperazine or metoclopramide can be combined with other antivertiginous medications. The patient with chronic recurrent vertigo usually is attempting to carry on normal activities and therefore sedation is undesirable. In this setting, meclizine, dimenhydrinate, and scopolamine are often useful. A major change in treatment strategy that has evolved over the past several years is to encourage patients to return to normal physical activity as rapidly as possible after an acute vertiginous attack.

> *Encourage patients to return to normal physical activity as soon as possible after an acute attack of vertigo.*

VESTIBULAR REHABILITATION

When the vestibular system has been permanently damaged, the initial state of imbalance at the level of the brain stem nuclei results in acute vertigo.[9] Gradually, the patient adapts to this imbalance through a process of compensation that requires intact vision and depth perception, normal proprioception in the neck and limbs, and intact sensation in the lower extremities. Central pathways are also integral to compensation, and damage to these areas results in a less effective recovery.

Clinicians have long been aware that vestibular compensation occurs more rapidly and is more complete if the patient begins exercising as soon as possible after a vestibular lesion. Controlled studies in primates have supported this general clinical observation. Baboons whose hind limbs were restrained by plaster casts after a unilateral vestibular lesion showed markedly delayed recovery of balance compared with lesioned animals that had been allowed normal motor exploration.[10] Visual experience is also necessary; lesioned animals kept in the light compensated faster than those kept in darkness.[11,12] Compensation is accelerated by stimulant drugs and slowed by sedation. For these reasons, vestibular exercise programs should be instituted as soon as possible after an injury to the vestibular system has been identified, and the use of sedating drugs and vestibular suppressants should be limited to the acute stage.

In addition to vertigo, vestibular lesions interfere with reflexes controlling eye movement during active head motion and with postural righting reflexes.[13] This interference can result in oscillopsia caused by head movements and a tendency to veer or fall to the side when walking. These symptoms and the associated dizziness can be improved by active exercises designed to speed compensation. Vestibular exercises should begin as soon as the acute stage of nausea and vomiting has ended and the underlying disease process is subsiding. Many of the exercises will result in dizziness. This sensation is a necessary stimulus for compensation; antivertiginous medications should be avoided during this

> *Active exercises can improve both dizziness and related symptoms such as oscillopsia.*

period to maximize the beneficial effect. Exercises should be done at least twice daily for several minutes but may be done as often as the patient can tolerate.

While nystagmus is present, the patient should attempt to focus the eyes and to move and hold them in the direction that provokes the most dizziness. Once the nystagmus diminishes to the point that a target can be "held" visually in all directions, the patient should begin eye and head coordination exercises. A useful exercise involves staring at a visual target while oscillating the head from side to side or up and down. The speed of the head movements can be gradually increased, as long as the target can be kept in good focus. Target changes using combined eye and head movements to jump quickly back and forth between two widely separated visual targets are also useful. Blinking during these fast head turns can help reduce symptoms of dizziness or visual blurring.

Once nystagmus diminishes, the patient should begin eye and head coordination exercises.

The patient should try to stand and walk while nystagmus is still present. It may be necessary to walk in contact with a wall or to use an assistant in the early stages. Slow, supported turns should be made initially. As improvement occurs, head movements should be added while standing and walking — at first, slow, side-to-side or up-and-down movements, then fast head turns in all directions. Learning to combine fast head turns with brief eye closure or blinks during walking turns can increase stability and decrease dizziness.[14]

Briefly closing the eyes or blinking can decrease dizziness from fast head turns.

Compensation requires from 2 to 6 months. Dizziness that persists beyond this time indicates either the presence of an ongoing, recurrent vestibular illness or poor compensation. The patient's history should be reviewed, and any vestibular suppressants should be discontinued. Evidence of central involvement or impairment of vision, proprioception, or sensation should be evaluated. If all areas are normal, no evidence of active disease is present, and no medications are in use, a program of habituation to dizziness should be instituted. All movements that provoke dizziness should be identified, and they should then be repeated as often as possible to maximize the symptom. This will gradually result in habituation to the provoking stimulus.

If dizziness persists beyond the time required for compensation and if no ongoing illness or reason for poor compensation is found, the patient should begin a program of habituation to dizziness, repeating provoking stimuli.

References

1. Foster CA, and Baloh RW: Drug therapy for vertigo. In Baloh RW, and Halmagyi GM (eds): Disorders of the Vestibular System. Oxford University Press, New York, 1996.
2. Mitchelson F: Pharmacologic agents affecting emesis: A review. Part I. Drugs 43:295, 1992.
3. Darlington CL, and Smith PF: What neurotransmitters are important in the vestibular system? In Baloh RW, and Halmagyi GM (eds): Disorders of the Vestibular System. Oxford University Press, New York, 1996.
4. Davis JR, Jennings RT, Beck BG, and Bagian JP: Treatment efficacy of intramuscular promethazine for space motion sickness. Aviat Space Environ Med 64:230, 1993.
5. Hasegawa S, Takeda N, Morita M, et al: Vestibular, central and gastral triggering of emesis: A study of individual susceptibility in rats. Acta Otolaryngol (Stockh) 112:927, 1992.

6. Ferrando SJ, and Eisendrath SJ: Adverse neuropsychiatric effects of dopamine antagonist medications. Psychosomatics 32:426, 1991.

7. Isah AO, Rawlins MD, and Bateman DN: Clinical pharmacology of prochlorperazine in healthy young males. Br J Clin Pharmacol 32:677, 1991.

8. Factor SA, and Matthews MK: Persistent extrapyramidal syndrome with dystonia and rigidity caused by combined metoclopramide and prochlorperazine. South Med J 84:626, 1991.

9. Curthoys IS, and Halmagyi GM: Vestibular compensation: A review of the oculomotor, neural and clinical consequences of unilateral vestibular loss. J Vestib Res 5:67, 1995.

10. Lacour M, Roll JP, and Appaix M: Modifications and development of spinal reflexes in the alert baboon (papio papio) following a unilateral vestibular neurotomy. Brain Res 113:255, 1976.

11. Igarashi M, Levy JK, O-Uchi T, et al.: Further study of physical exercise and locomotor balance compensation after unilateral labyrinthectomy in squirrel monkeys. Acta Otolaryngol (Stockh) 92:101, 1981.

12. Igarashi M, Ishikawa K, Ishii M, et al.: Physical exercise and balance compensation after total ablation of vestibular organs. Prog Brain Res 76:395, 1988.

13. Herdman SJ: Vestibular rehabilitation. In Baloh RW, and Halmagyi GM (eds): Disorders of the Vestibular System. Oxford University Press, New York, 1996.

14. Foster CA, and Baloh RW: Episodic vertigo. In Rakel RE (ed): Conn's Current Therapy. W. B. Saunders, Philadelphia, 1995.

12

Symptomatic Treatment of Tinnitus

Chapter Outline

GENERAL CONSIDERATIONS

Tinnitus is a symptom, not a disease. As in the case of vertigo, whenever a specific cause can be identified, it should be treated. Unfortunately, the cause often cannot be found, and even when a cause is found and treated, tinnitus may persist. Symptomatic management may then be the only option.

Most patients with tinnitus can be helped by a detailed interview together with the relevant examination and laboratory investigations (see Chapter 9), followed by reassurance, where this can be given. Often exacerbating factors such as chronic anxiety and depression can be identified. A "vicious cycle" develops whereby the state of mind makes the tinnitus worse and the tinnitus in turn makes the anxiety and depression worse. The patient may become preoccupied with the tinnitus to the exclusion of all else, feeling that the tinnitus makes life not worth living. Some may even attempt suicide. The elderly are particularly vulnerable to this problem, since they often have fewer activities to occupy their time. Psychological therapy is typically directed toward decreasing the level of annoyance associated with the tinnitus rather than decreasing its perceived loudness (Fig. 85).[1] In the severely depressed patient, supportive psychotherapy and antidepressant drugs can help to improve the quality of life and reduce the effect of the tinnitus.[2-4] The American Tinnitus Association provides a good opportunity for patients to meet fellow sufferers, thereby

> *If the cause of tinnitus cannot be found, or if the tinnitus persists after treatment, symptomatic management may be required.*

> *Reassurance or psychological therapy directed at decreasing the level of annoyance may reduce the effect of tinnitus.*

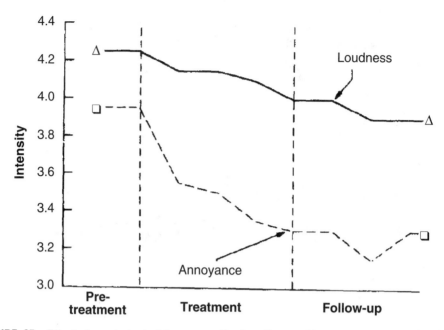

FIGURE 85 Effect of psychological therapy on tinnitus distress. Mean values for ratings of loudness (Δ) and for annoyance (□) during the pretreatment orientation period, throughout treatment, and during the 3-month follow-up. Annoyance ratings declined significantly but loudness ratings did not. Scales ranged from 1 = very soft/not at all annoying, to 7 = the loudest ever/the most annoying. (Reprinted from Behav Res Ther 24: Jakes, SC, et al: The effects of reassurance, relaxation training, and distraction on chronic tinnitus sufferers. p. 501, 1986, with kind permission from Elsevier Science, Ltd., The Boulevard, Langford Lane, Kidlington OX5 1GB, UK.)

If patients hear more ambient noise, they are often less aware of their tinnitus.

Common substances worsen tinnitus in some patients.

providing group support and keeping patients informed of progress in the field.

Patients with both hearing loss and tinnitus may benefit from a hearing aid, not only for improved communication, but also because amplification of the ambient sound may effectively mask the tinnitus. This mechanism probably explains the frequent observation that removal of cerumen from the external auditory canal improves tinnitus. When the ear wax is removed, the patient hears ambient noise normally and is less aware of the tinnitus. When cerumen is attached to the tympanic membrane, tinnitus may result from local mechanical effects on the conduction system. For patients who find their tinnitus most obtrusive when trying to sleep, a bedside FM clock radio tuned between stations can provide an effective masking sound that will switch itself off after the patient falls asleep.

As indicated in Chapter 9, numerous drugs can produce or aggravate tinnitus. A careful drug history should be taken and a drug-free trial period considered when possible. Some patients notice that caffeine, alcohol, or nicotine exacerbates their tinnitus, and they experience significant relief when these drugs are discontinued. Occasionally, occult food additives, such as quinine in tonic water and bitter lemon, can be identified as the cause of tinnitus.

RELAXATION TECHNIQUES

A wide range of relaxation techniques have been used to treat tinnitus, including biofeedback, hypnotherapy, and acupuncture.[5-7] **Biofeedback** has been most extensively evaluated, although for obvious reasons controlled studies are lacking.[8,9] As with psychological therapy in general, the goal of biofeedback is to help the patient cope with the tinnitus rather than to reduce its intensity. Generally, biofeedback training involves giving the subject feedback about a physiological variable to be controlled (e.g., blood pressure or heart rate) and the subject's task is to learn to produce the desired changes in that variable through any means available. Because tinnitus is typically not detectable by external sensors, however, there is no way to provide feedback to the patient about the loudness of the tinnitus, so when biofeedback is used to treat tinnitus, it is used as a means for relaxation rather than as a specific method for reducing the loudness of tinnitus. Patients are typically given feedback from electromyographic recordings in muscles, usually the frontalis muscle, with the assumption that reducing muscular tension will reduce stress and anxiety, which will in turn allow the tinnitus sufferer to cope with the symptom better. Biofeedback is often better accepted by patients with tinnitus than more formal psychological counseling sessions or psychotherapy.

Biofeedback training is used to teach patients to reduce muscular tension, thereby lowering stress and enabling them to cope better with their tinnitus.

MASKING TECHNIQUES

Many patients prefer hearing an external noise (a **masking sound**) to their own tinnitus. The masking sound may be preferable to tinnitus because it can be more easily ignored. If the patient is not profoundly deaf, it is often possible to generate a sound sufficiently loud to make the patient oblivious to his or her tinnitus. Although the idea of masking with an external sound dates back to the time of Hippocrates, tinnitus maskers have only recently been developed and evaluated. These devices are small sound generators that can be worn behind the ear, similar to a hearing aid. The bandwidth of the masking noise is tailored to the patient's tinnitus. Hearing amplification and masking can be combined in some units, so that patients with significant hearing loss and tinnitus may also be helped by masking.

The bandwidth of the noise generated by a tinnitus masker is tailored to each patient's tinnitus.

As a general rule, the effectiveness of tinnitus masking is inversely proportional to the loudness of the masking sound required.[10] Thus, the first step in fitting a masking unit is to identify a sound that effectively masks the tinnitus at the lowest sensation level. Tones or noise bands covering the patient's usable hearing range are presented using an ascending series of sound levels separated by intervals of 2 dB to determine the minimum sensation level required to provide complete masking of the tinnitus. In this way the minimum masking level is determined at each frequency, so that the most effective region of the frequency scale is identified.

One dramatic result of tinnitus masking is the production of **residual inhibition,** the suppression of tinnitus for a variable duration after the masking sound is removed. Residual inhibition occurs in most patients, but unfortunately it usually lasts only a brief time. To test for residual inhibition, a masking stimulus is presented at the minimum masking level plus 10 dB for 1 minute, and the patient is asked to describe the tinnitus when the masking sound is turned off.[10] If the masking stimulus is a good match for the tinnitus, most patients (about 75%) will report that their tinnitus is either gone or markedly diminished. The tinnitus usually returns gradually to its pretest level in less than 1 minute. Rarely, residual inhibition will last for several hours after 1 minute of masking. The degree of residual inhibition with this simple 1-minute test gives some indication of the efficacy and success of long-term masking.

Follow-up studies to assess the efficacy of tinnitus masking units have produced variable results. In one study, only 9 of 34 patients who were considered candidates for masking units reported that they were receiving some form of relief from their tinnitus.[11] In another study, only 10 of 31 patients who rented masking units purchased instruments after a 30-day period, and only 2 of these were using their instruments on a regular basis.[12] The most extensive experience with tinnitus maskers has been accumulated by the group at the University of Oregon in Portland.[10,13] Over the 3-year period from 1976 through 1978, 493 patients were seen at the tinnitus clinic and, of these, 380 were advised to be fitted with one of three instruments: a masking device, a hearing aid, or a combined masking device and hearing aid (**tinnitus instrument**). In those cases in which an instrument was not recommended, the tinnitus could not be effectively masked or patients indicated that the masking sound was not an acceptable substitute for their tinnitus. Of the 380 patients for whom an instrument was recommended, 158 (42%) were still wearing the instrument after a period ranging from 1 to 3 years (Table 23). Of the 216 patients who actually purchased instruments, 73% were still using them. Of note, 45% of the patients reported that they received total or partial relief of their tinnitus when wearing a hearing aid alone, without any additional masking. Very few patients (6%) obtained complete relief of their tinnitus with any of the devices.

Erlandsson et al.[14] compared the effect of a tinnitus masker to a placebo device in 17 patients with severe tinnitus. The placebo device looked exactly like the masking device, and the patients were told that the two types of equipment exerted their assumed effects on tinnitus in different ways, one by emitting sounds and the other by weak electrical stimulation. Patients rated their tinni-

After masking, most patients experience a period of suppression of their tinnitus, called residual inhibition.

Follow-up studies to assess the efficacy of tinnitus masking units have produced variable results.

Table 23   Tinnitus Masking Program: Follow-Up Results*

	No. % Maskers		No. % Hearing Aids		No. % Tinnitus Instruments		No. % Totals	
Recommended for *Trial Purchase*	204		132		44		380	
Purchased device	93	46	91	69	32	73	216	57
Currently wearing device	61	30 (66)†	68	52 (75)	29	66 (91)	158	42 (73)
Tried device but did not purchase	58	28	17	13	5	11	80	37
Duration Wearing Unit								
Less than 1 yr	37	40	24	26	12	38	73	34
Less than 2 yr	43	43	32	39	12	38	87	40
More than 2 yr	13	14	35	39	8	24	56	26
Relief								
Total	6	6	2	2	2	16	13	6
Partial	69	74	39	43	22	68	130	60
None	18	19	50	55	5	16	73	34

*Results of follow-up survey of 380 tinnitus patients who were provided specific recommendations to participate in the masking program at the University of Oregon, Portland.

†Numbers in parentheses = percentages of those patients who purchased instruments and are currently wearing them.

Adapted from Schleuning AJ, Johnson RM, and Vernon JA: Evaluation of a tinnitus masking program: A follow-up study of 598 patients. Ear Hear 1:71, 1980, with permission.

tus intensity during a baseline period, during treatment with the portable masker, and during a period with the comparable placebo apparatus. Group analysis showed no significant differences between any of the three periods. Seven patients showed significantly reduced tinnitus intensity ratings during the masking period, and five reported decreased intensity with the placebo. Although the study is relatively small, it does raise questions regarding the mechanism of action of masking devices—specifically, whether there is some direct effect on the pathophysiology of tinnitus or whether it is simply another form of psychological therapy.

HABITUATION THERAPY

Jastreboff and colleagues have developed a treatment for tinnitus based on the goal of removing the perception of tinnitus from the patient's consciousness by initiating and facilitating the process of tinnitus **habituation**.[15,16] According to their behavioral retraining theory, masking is actually counterproductive because for habituation to occur the stimulus being habituated must be perceived during the training period. They often use a white-noise stimulus but not with the goal of masking the tinnitus. Instead, their goal is to make the detection of the tinnitus-related signal more difficult, thus facilitating the process of habituation. They argue that whether tinnitus can or cannot be totally masked has no relevance for predicting the outcome of their habituation therapy. In cases where there is a hearing impairment, appropriately fitted hearing aids can also be useful.

The goal of habituation therapy is to remove the perception of tinnitus from the patient's consciousness.

Patients are managed by a multidisciplinary team of otologist, audiologist, and psychologist with the ultimate goal of removing the perception of tinnitus from the patient's consciousness. The team uses cognitive therapy with highly specific and directive counseling while decreasing detectability of the tinnitus by introducing a low-level neutral acoustic signal such as white noise. They report that this process typically takes from 12 to 18 months to reach a level where most patients are not aware of their tinnitus most of the time. At this stage, the white-noise generators are not needed any longer and many patients discontinue their use. From time to time, particularly at periods of increased stress, tinnitus resurfaces, but a short repetition of the treatment for a few weeks is usually sufficient to restore the patient to the previous level of comfort. Although reported results are impressive, they will need to be reproduced by others before such an expensive treatment program can be recommended for broader use.

DRUGS

Many investigators have reported relief of some types of tinnitus with intravenous lidocaine.[17-19] The mechanism of action of lidocaine is uncertain; it probably affects both the peripheral and central auditory pathways. Tinnitus that accompanies middle ear disease is not affected by lidocaine. Typically, a maximum dose of 2 mg/kg body weight in 1% solution is given intravenously over 3 to 4 minutes. In those patients who experience some relief (approximately 60% of patients with tinnitus), relief lasts between 10 and 30 minutes, but occasionally it lasts as long as several days. Although not a practical long-term treatment for tinnitus, the experience with lidocaine provides grounds for optimism that a similar drug might be found that would have prolonged bioavailability when given orally.

The tinnitus relief provided to many patients by lidocaine has prompted research into possible drug therapies for tinnitus.

Because of the known anticonvulsant effect of lidocaine, several anticonvulsants have been tried in the treatment of tinnitus.[18,20,21] Most work has been done with carbamazepine, but in spite of some encouraging initial reports, this drug has now been largely abandoned in the routine treatment of subjective tinnitus. Because of bothersome side effects, it should be reserved for patients with intractable severe tinnitus who have dramatic response to intravenous lidocaine. To minimize side effects, the recommended treatment regimen is to begin with 100 mg at night and then add an extra 100 mg daily each week until the patient is taking 200 mg 3 times a day, at which time the serum concentration is checked and dosage adjusted.[21] The only double-blind placebo-controlled study of carbamazepine found no significant difference between the drug and placebo, but unfortunately the study included patients whose tinnitus showed no response to lidocaine.[22]

Phenytoin, barbiturates, and sodium valproate have also been used with varying success in treating intractable tinnitus.[21]

A number of drugs that are chemically allied with lidocaine are being developed and tested. Controlled clinical trials comparing these drugs with placebos are needed before their role in the management of tinnitus can be determined.

ELECTRICAL STIMULATION

As part of the recent interest in stimulating the ears of deaf patients electrically, it was observed that positive current could evoke a "silence" sensation in patients with tinnitus.[23,24] Brackmann noted that stimulation of a cochlear implant can reduce or eliminate contralateral as well as ipsilateral tinnitus and that the implantation operation itself reduced or eliminated preexisting tinnitus in about 80% of a small sample of 29 patients.[25]

Others have noted that tinnitus can sometimes be abolished through the transtympanic application of brief electrical pulses to the cochlea. With this technique, electrical stimulation is effective in suppressing only tinnitus clearly localized in the ipsilateral ear; it has no effect on tinnitus in the contralateral ear. Cazals, Negrevergne, and Aran felt that the electrical stimulation with positive pulses produces the equivalent of hyperpolarization in the neural elements of the cochlea and its central projections.[26] This does not explain why pulses of current are effective but steady-state stimulation usually is not, nor why there is a critical "frequency" of pulse stimulations. This procedure could have obvious risks that have not yet been assessed relative to potential benefits. Although it is worthy of further investigation, safety is a concern and has yet to be compared with other, less invasive methods of treatment.

The technique of suppressing tinnitus by applying electrical pulses to the cochlea is still being studied.

SURGERY

Surgical treatment of tinnitus has been generally disappointing. Even patients who have undergone removal of acoustic neuromas or successful stapedectomies for otosclerosis report variable changes in their tinnitus. In a series of 500 patients who had acoustic neuromas removed, 83% had tinnitus before surgery and in 11% tinnitus was the initial symptom.[27] A postoperative survey revealed that tinnitus was improved in 40%, worse in 50%, and unchanged in the remaining 10%. In patients with otosclerosis whose chief complaint is tinnitus, the tinnitus frequently worsens despite a successful stapedectomy; if the stapedectomy is unsuccessful, the tinnitus often becomes unbearable.[28] For these reasons, stapedectomy should not be offered as treatment for tinnitus in patients with otosclerosis.

Even when a lesion can be localized to the inner ear or cochlear nerve, removing these structures often has little effect on

Surgical treatment of subjective tinnitus is seldom successful.

Surgery can cure objective tinnitus caused by a vascular malformation or tumor in the mastoid.

the tinnitus. Apparently once the tinnitus is initiated, it is propagated in the central auditory pathways and no longer relies on a peripheral generator.

A single exception to the generally dismal record of surgical treatment of tinnitus is complete cure of objective tinnitus after surgical correction of a vascular malformation or tumor in the mastoid.

References

1. Jakes SC, Hallam RS, Rachman S, and Hinchcliffe R: The effects of reassurance, relaxation training and distracting on chronic tinnitus sufferers. Behav Res Ther 24:497, 1986.
2. Sullivan MD, Dobie RA, Sakai CS, and Katon WJ: Treatment of depressed tinnitus patients with nortriptyline. Ann Otol Rhinol Laryngol 98:867, 1989.
3. Dobie RA, Sullivan MD, Katon WL, et al.: Antidepressant treatment of tinnitus patients. Interim report of a randomized clinical trial. Acta Otolaryngol (Stockh) 112:242, 1992.
4. Mihail RC, Crowley JM, Walden BE, et al.: The tricyclic trimipramine in the treatment of subjective tinnitus. Ann Otol Rhinol Larylgol 97:120, 1988.
5. Ireland CE, Wilson PH, Tonkin JP, and Platt-Hepworth S: An evaluation of relaxation training in the treatment of tinnitus. Behav Res Ther 23:423, 1985.
6. Marks NJ, Karle H, and Onisiphorou C: A controlled trial of hypnotherapy in tinnitus. Clin Otolaryngol 10:43, 1985.
7. Mann F: Acupuncture in auditory and related disorders. Br J Audiol 8:23, 1974.
8. Grossan M: Treatment of subjective tinnitus with biofeedback. Ear Nose Throat J 55:22, 1976.
9. House JW: Treatment of severe tinnitus with biofeedback training. Laryngoscope 88:406, 1978.
10. Vernon JA, and Meikle MB: Tinnitus masking: Unresolved problems. In Tinnitus, Ciba Foundation Symposium. Pitman Books, London, 1981.
11. Roeser RJ, and Price DR: Clinical experience with tinnitus maskers. Ear Hear 1:63, 1980.
12. Rose DE: Tinnitus maskers: A follow-up. Ear Hear 1:69, 1980.
13. Schleuning AJ, Johnson RM, and Vernon JA: Evaluation of a tinnitus masking program: A follow-up study of 598 patients. Ear Hear 1:71, 1980.
14. Erlandsson S, Ringdahl A, Hutchins T, and Carlsson SG: Treatment of tinnitus: A controlled comparison of masking and placebo. Br J Audiol 21:37, 1987.
15. Jastreboff PJ: Phantom auditory perception (tinnitus): Mechanisms of generation and perception. Neurosci Res 8:221, 1990.
16. Jastreboff PJ, and Hazell JWP: A neurophysiological approach to tinnitus: Clinical implications. Br J Audiol 27:7, 1993.
17. Melding PS, Goodey RJ, and Thorne PR: The use of intravenous lidocaine in the diagnosis and treatment of tinnitus. J Laryngol Otol 92:115, 1978.
18. Shea JJ, and Harell M: Management of tinnitus aurium with lidocaine and carbamazepine. Laryngoscope 88:1477, 1978.
19. Duckert LG, and Rees TS: Treatment of tinnitus with intravenous lidocaine: A double-blind randomized trial. Otolaryngol Head Neck Surg 91:550, 1983.
20. Melding PS, and Goodey RJ: The treatment of tinnitus with oral anticonvulsants. J Laryngol Otol 93:111, 1979.
21. Goodey RJ: Drugs in the treatment of tinnitus. In Tinnitus, Ciba Foundation Symposium. Pitman Books, London, 1981.
22. Donaldson I: Tegretol: A double blind trial in tinnitus. J Laryngol Otol 95:947, 1981.
23. Portmann M, Cazals Y, Negrevergne M, and Aran J-M: Temporary tinnitus suppression in man through electrical stimulation of the cochlea. Acta Otolaryngol (Stockh) 87:294, 1979.
24. Aran J, and Cazals Y: Electrical suppression of tinnitus. In Tinnitus, Ciba Foundation Symposium. Pitman Books, London, 1981.

25. Brackmann DE: Panel discussion. In Shulman A (Chairman): Tinnitus: Proceedings of the First International Tinnitus Seminar. J Laryngol Otol Suppl 4:143, 1981.
26. Cazals Y, Negrevergne M, and Aran J-M: Electrical stimulation of the cochlea in man: Hearing induction and tinnitus suppression. J Am Audiol Soc 3:200, 1978.
27. House JW, and Brackmann DE: Tinnitus: Surgical treatment. In Tinnitus, Ciba Foundation Symposium. Pitman Books, London, 1981.
28. Goodhill V: Ear Diseases, Deafness and Dizziness. Harper and Row, Hagerstown MD, 1979.

Index